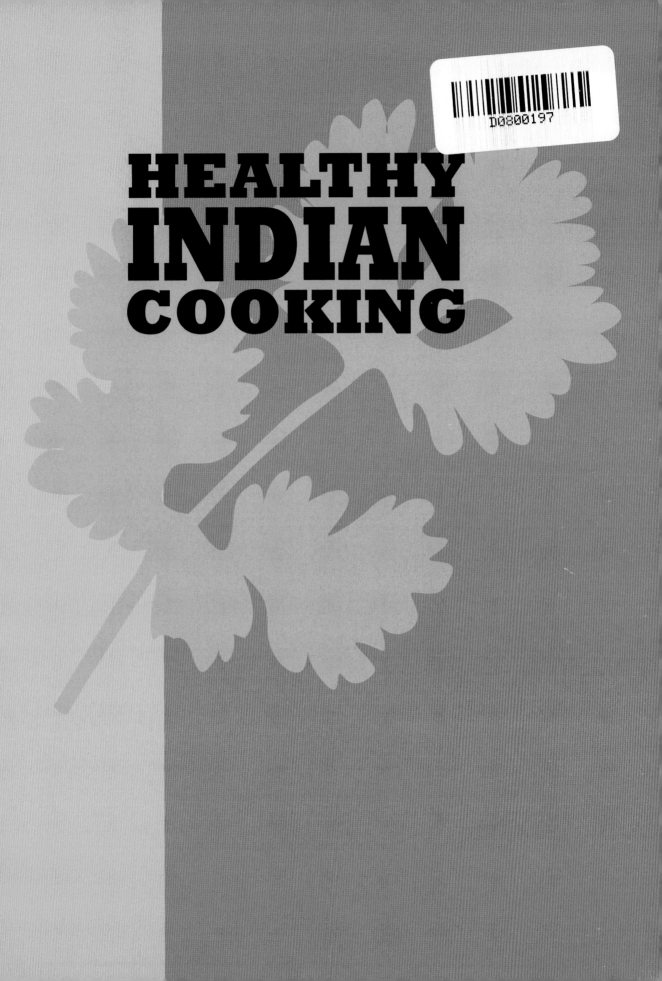

HEALTHY INDIAN COOKING

THIS IS A CARLTON BOOK

Text copyright © 2003 Monisha Bharadwaj
Design copyright © 2003 Carlton Books Limited

This edition published in 2013 by
Carlton Books Limited
20 Mortimer Street
London W1T 3JW

10 9 8 7 6 5 4 3 2 1

A CIP catalogue record for this book
is available from the British Library.

ISBN 978-1-78097-263-3

Printed and bound in Dubai

ABOUT THE RECIPES
All recipes in this book are for four people. Menu suggestions are
precisely that. I have merely provided them as a guide to inspire you
to experiment for yourself. After all, Ayurvedic nutrition is all about
eating what makes you, as an individual, feel healthy and happy, both
in the short term and throughout your life.

The information and recipes in this book are not intended to diagnose,
treat or cure. This book is not a substitute for professional medical
advice. If in doubt, please consult your doctor as soon as possible.

HEALTHY INDIAN COOKING

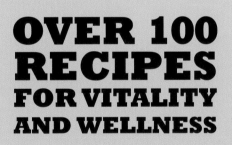

OVER 100 RECIPES
FOR VITALITY
AND WELLNESS

Monisha Bharadwaj

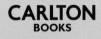

CARLTON
BOOKS

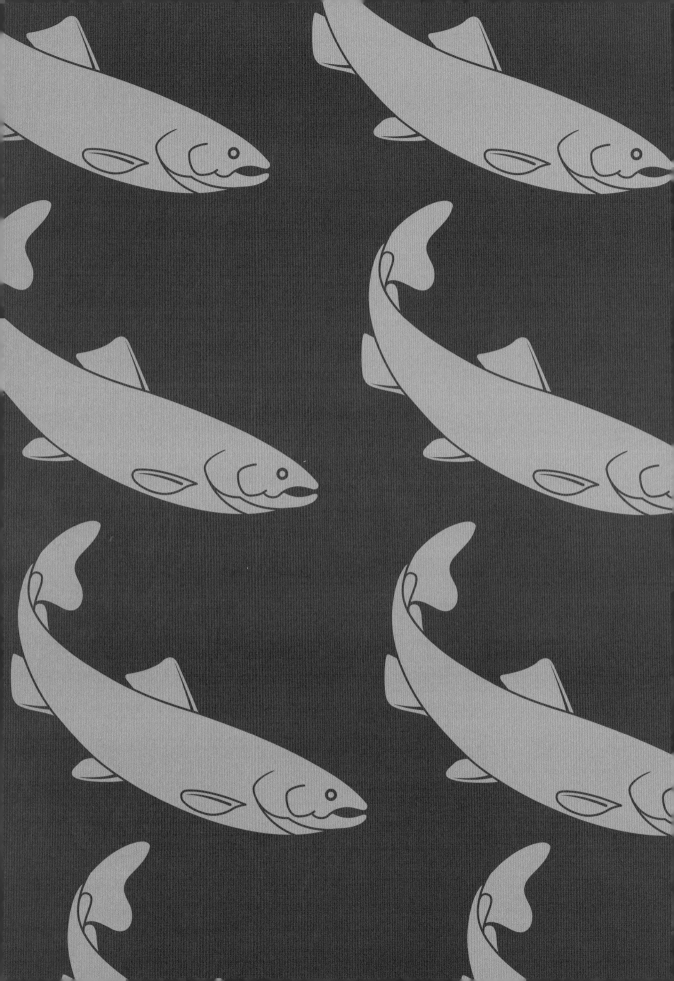

Contents

Introduction

It is widely recognized today that what we eat affects our health, mood, energy levels and entire outlook on life. More and more people are turning towards healthier eating options such as organic foods, a larger proportion of fruits and vegetables in their daily diet and unprocessed foods rather than refined ones. In this fast-paced age, stress, ill health, anger and eventual burnout are common, all of which are exacerbated by unhealthy eating. Today we all want to eat delicious food that will make us feel fit, healthy and vibrant. We are choosing foods that will make our skin glow, our hair shine and our bodies strong. Good health and a feeling of being at peace with oneself have become primary guiding factors when we select what we eat.

Contrary to popular belief outside India, everyday Indian cooking is not unhealthy or fattening. In fact, it is a high-energy cuisine that has always subscribed to natural and whole foods such as wholemeal (whole-wheat) flour rather than white flour or raw cane sugar over refined white sugar, for example.

Along with eating the right foods, Indians also believe that peaceful surroundings and a quiet mind at mealtimes help to boost immunity, aid digestion and conserve stamina for whatever lies ahead. Food is not meant to be eaten on the run or when you are distracted.

Also, cooking methods must preserve the *prana*, or life force, of food. Overcooking, long periods of freezing and adding preservatives all effectively kill prana and make food unwholesome. Ayurvedic nutrition takes all this and more into account.

Ayurvedic Wisdom

The basis of Indian cookery is a treasury of ayurvedic wisdom. Ayurveda is seen as a complete way of life, designed to enhance health, a general sense of wellbeing and longevity. It was developed thousands of years ago by Himalayan sages who used natural herbs, seeds, leaves, flowers, fruits and barks to heal and nourish. This holistic system of natural medicine is gentle and has few side effects, and it is therefore becoming increasingly popular all over the world. The cures address the root of the ailment, rather than just the symptoms, and thus work in the long term as well as the short. Ayurveda is all about the intrinsic links between your mental, spiritual and physical wellbeing and taking a holistic approach to your health.

The Five Elements

Ayurveda is based largely on the principle that all creation is made up of the five elements: air, fire, water, earth and ether. These elements exist in nature, in food and even within our bodies. Air promotes health; fire is purification; water signifies movement and fluidity; earth symbolizes energy and fecundity; and ether, or space, echoes with vibrations of the Divine. When all the elements are maintained in harmonious balance in our bodies, good health naturally follows.

According to ayurveda, good health can be achieved first by nourishing the *dhatus*, or seven major kinds of tissues, including the muscles, fat and bony tissue. Secondly, the body needs to be cleansed of *ama*, or the metabolic waste that accumulates in the body due to poor digestion or malabsorption. These days, ama has also come to mean the harmful effects of pollution caused by a modern way of living.

Satmya and Okasatmya

In ayurveda *satmya* is anything that is beneficial to the body and mind, even long after it has been consumed. *Okasatmya*, on the other hand, is a concept explaining how a certain diet or lifestyle becomes nonharmful to the body through regular use and exposure. If, for instance, your ancestors have eaten large amounts of cholesterol-laden red meat and if you, too, have eaten it for most of your life, you will almost certainly be able to metabolize it with fewer ill effects than someone who has suddenly taken a fancy to eating red meat every day but has no history of having eaten it before.

According to your individual constitution and history, something that works for you may be a slow road to ill-health for someone else. After all, one man's meat is another man's poison.

Your Constitution

Ayurveda refers to the unique combination of energy present in each individual at birth as *prakruti*, that person's constitution. The proportion and balance of the five elements in your body determines your prakruti, and therefore no two people are exactly alike. Unlike Western beliefs in which general rules such as eating five portions of fruits or vegetables a day are popular, the ayurveda principle believes that there is no general path to health and that each person must be treated individually, depending on his or her prakruti.

The three basic constitutions are determined by energies called *doshas*. These are *vata* (governed by the elements of air and ether), *pitta* (governed by fire and water) and *kapha* (governed by water and earth). If you understand the particular needs of your prakruti, or constitution, and choose foods as well as a lifestyle accordingly, you give yourself the best chance of good health. Sometimes two doshas form a combination in a single individual, usually with one of the doshas predominating. Rarely, all three of the doshas are present equally, making it a balanced, or tridoshic, constitution.

The balance of the doshas within your body is affected by the environment in which you live; the climate and season of the year, or even the time of the day; and also the foods that you eat and when. Each dosha possesses dominant traits or characteristics, and the following guidelines should point to whether you are a vata, a pitta or a kapha, or perhaps a combination of any two of the doshas.

Vata

- You are lean and tend to be either unusually tall or unusually short.
- A lack of good muscle tone means that you are unable to do heavy physical work, and you find it difficult to put on weight.
- Your skin is dry, your hair rough and kinky, and your hands and feet are often cold.
- Your voice is high-pitched.
- Although you are creative, you change your mind easily.
- You suffer from constipation, brittle nails and perspire little.
- You prefer a warm, sunny climate, have a variable appetite, dislike routine and love to be physically active.
- You dream often (of flying, moving, jumping), but do not remember your dreams.
- You have a tendency to snack often, and you sleep lightly.
- When you become stressed, you veer towards fear or anxiety.
- Your sex drive is variable, but your fantasies are vivid.
- You are quite a spendthrift.

Pitta

- You are of medium build and well proportioned.
- You lose or gain weight easily, and have a good appetite and metabolism.
- You need frequent meals and rarely suffer from constipation.
- Your skin and hair are oily and fine, and you prefer a cool climate.
- Creative and competitive, you are also intellectual and have strong opinions.
- You become angry and frustrated when stressed and are vehement about putting across your point of view.
- You sleep well.
- Your sex drive is high and, if left unfulfilled, you quickly become angry and moody.
- You perspire freely, your hands are warm and you are frequently thirsty.
- You make an excellent leader and are good at setting routines.

Kapha

- You are robust in build and have heavy bones.
- You gain weight easily, but conversely find losing it difficult.
- Your skin is thick and cool, and you tan only slowly, if at all.
- Your hair is thick and wavy.
- You prefer a dry climate and are comfortable in hot or cold weather.
- Regular bowel movements, a good appetite and a normal digestion are not affected by your love of fatty, starchy foods.
- You love leisure activities, sleep particularly soundly and often dream of water and rivers.
- You are generally calm and placid.
- Your opinions and ideas are slow to change, and you tend to avoid difficult situations.
- When you are ill, you tend to retain fluid or produce a lot of mucus.
- Your sex drive is steady, and your voice is pleasant and well modulated.

Ayurvedic Nutrition

According to ayurvedic principles all foods consist of six tastes (*rasa*); two potencies (*veerya*), or the properties of being cooling or heating to the body; and three postdigestive long-term effects on the body (*vipaka*), that is, whether they aggravate or ameliorate a particular dosha.

Taste

The word *rasa* has many meanings in Sanskrit. It denotes emotion as well as taste. Taste has a profound effect on our physical and mental health. Ayurveda recommends food combinations and cooking styles to enhance the tastes that promote good health and remedy specific ailments. There are six tastes in ayurveda: sweet, sour, salty, pungent, bitter and astringent. All of these have specific effects on the doshas and subsequently your physical and mental wellbeing.

Sweet

This taste is universally accepted by all of the doshas and is the most beneficial of all the tastes. It has a cooling veerya and tends to be heavy and moist. In moderation it is extremely satisfying and, emotionally, it promotes a feeling of wellbeing.

Sour

The veerya, or potency, of sour is heating and therefore this taste promotes digestive fire, or *agni*, in our systems. Sour foods tend to be mildly heavy and moist. Emotionally, an excess of this taste can cause envy or 'sourpuss' negativity.

Salty

This comprises water and fire, which give it its heating attribute. Its long-term effect is moistening, and therefore people who eat too much salt will be prone to water retention. They can also seem too rigid in their behaviour.

Pungent

This taste is the one most stimulating to the digestion. Its qualities are light and dry.

Bitter

As found in some leafy greens, a bitter taste is cold, dry and light. Consuming bitter tastes helps to balance all the others.

Astringent

An astringent taste is slightly light and dry, and has a cooling veerya. This taste hampers digestion and it is associated with a detached attitude to life.

'Cooling' and 'Heating' Foods

Ayurveda refers to digestive power as fire (agni). Too much food, foods that are cooling, and heavy or processed foods rapidly put out this fire, whereas too little food does not provide enough kindling. Most Indians are taught in childhood about the heating and cooling qualities of different foods, and how they affect the body during the various seasons. Summers are meant for cooling foods such as milk, coconut and fennel. Winters are for warming foods such as honey, red lentils and most spices. It is best to experiment with various foods to see their effect on your body.

EIGHT RULES OF AN AYURVEDIC DIET

1 Prakruti
Choose a combination of foods depending on their nature, i.e. their inherent heaviness or lightness, and your particular constitution. For instance, meat is quite heavy to digest, while vegetables are light.

2 Karana
The processing of foods affects their influence on our bodies. Generally, cooked foods are easier to digest, with the exception of fruits and some vegetables. Frying adds heaviness, whereas stir-frying helps to introduce a degree of lightness into food. Microwave cooking destroys prana and is not recommended.

3 Samyoga
Always combine foods healthily and never mix contrary foods. For example, fish and dairy foods should not be combined, as they each require a different rate of acid secretion as well as differing acid concentrations for proper digestion.

4 Rashi
Control the quantity of food that you eat according to your individual constitution.

5 Desha
Eat according to your environment. Consider the seasons and factors such as humidity and pollution.

6 Kala
Pay attention to the time at which you eat. Eat only when the previous meal has had a chance to be properly digested and avoid eating too late in the day.

7 Upayoga sanstha
Follow the golden rules of eating. Eat food when it is hot if it is meant to be hot. Concentrate on the act of eating rather than on watching television, reading or other distractions. Be calm and unhurried. Do not smoke and try not to drink too much during a meal.

8 Upabhokta
Choose what you eat depending on how you feel. Listen to your body and never force yourself to eat or consume food or drink against your instincts.

COLOUR THERAPY

In India the influence of colours on our physical and emotional wellbeing was recognized thousands of years ago. Nature itself was the original inspiration. A blue sea felt calming, an orange sunrise created joy and a green forest was rejuvenating.

Human beings are composed of several colour vibrations, and we respond to colour physically and emotionally at every moment of our lives. Factors such as our lifestyle, diet and a fluctuating emotional state can all contribute to an imbalance in our health. According to colour therapy these factors can result in there being either an overdose or perhaps too little of a particular colour in our body's energy centres. When the colour energies in our bodies are in balance, however, we feel healthy and vibrant.

So how are colours absorbed into the body? Each of us has a set of energy centres in our bodies known as *chakras*. Seven of these are considered to be the most important, and these chakras are connected to the body's nerve centres. They are also associated with certain colours:

- **Muladhara chakra (base of the spine)**
  – absorbs red energy

- **Swadhishthana chakra (small of the back)**
  – absorbs orange energy

- **Manipura chakra (lumbar region)**
  – absorbs yellow energy

- **Anahata chakra (heart)**
  – absorbs green energy

- **Vishuddha chakra (near the throat)**
  – absorbs blue energy

- **Ajna chakra (between the eyebrows)**
  – absorbs indigo energy

- **Sahasrara chakra (above the crown of the head)**
  – absorbs violet energy

The energy ray of each of the recipes included in this book is indicated by the page's background colour.

GLOSSARY OF AYURVEDIC TERMS

Acharya Charak Author of the *Charak Samhita*, an ancient and respected ayurvedic textbook that is still referred to today.

agni The sacred Hindu god of fire, signifying purification, and also the term for digestive fire. If your metabolism is slow or sluggish, you are considered to have low agni. It is also possible for too much agni to be present in your system.

ama Internal bodily toxins which are created as a result of incomplete digestion or elimination, or an unhealthy metabolism.

ayurveda An ancient Indian science of holistic healing and herbal medicine aimed at maintaining physical, mental and spiritual wellbeing.

chakra A vital energy centre of the body.

dhatu One of the seven basic tissues of the body.

dosha The biological energy that determines individual constitution: vata, pitta and kapha are the three energies, or doshas. All foods are considered to have particular effects on the doshas, which is why some foods are suitable for particular people, but not for others.

kapha One of the three doshas, made up of the elements of earth and water.

ojas The essential energy of the body.

okasatmya An unbalanced diet that has become nonharmful to the body through habitual use.

panchakarma The five purifying practices of ayurveda aimed at detoxification.

pitta One of the three doshas, made up of the elements of fire and water.

prakruti Our innate nature; also our biological constitution at birth.

prana The breath of life, or vital life force, present in every living thing.

prithvi The element of earth.

rajas The quality of energy and action.

rasa Taste – there are considered to be six basic rasas in ayurveda. The word is also used to mean plasma, or feeling and emotion.

sattvic The quality of being calming and balancing. Considered a positive attribute.

shita Cool.

slakshna Slimy.

snigdha Oily.

tamasic The quality of being resistant and inert.

tridoshic A balanced state in which the three doshas – vata, pitta and kapha – are all present. A tridoshic constitution is one in which an individual possesses the three doshas in equilibrium. Tridoshic food is suited to all the constitutions.

ushna Hot.

vata One of the three doshas, made up of the elements of ether and air.

vayu The element of air.

Vedas The four ancient Hindu scriptures of India, the *Rig Veda*, *Sama Veda*, *Atharva Veda* and *Yajur Veda*, which contain hymns, poems and rituals.

veerya The effect of a particular food on the body's digestion, especially its action of being either heating or cooling.

vipaka The postdigestive effect of a food.

viruddhashana Forbidden food combinations as proscribed by ayurveda.

The Basics

You really do not need much to start cooking healthy Indian food in your home. I tend to stock key spices and herbs, and buy small amounts for specific recipes when I need them. This ensures that I use fresh, flavourful ingredients each time.

Also, I dislike a cluttered kitchen filled with specialized and often rarely used equipment. My list of essential equipment, which is given below, which has seen me through years of cooking.

- A few heavy-bottomed saucepans to withstand intense cooking processes such as deep-frying.
- A couple of *kadhais*, or Indian 'woks'. The shape and thickness of these cooking pans ensures even cooking, and they can be successfully used for either deep-frying or stir-frying.
- A food processor or blender – no Indian kitchen is complete without this. It is used to grind herbs, spices, nuts and fruits to a smooth mixture that forms the base of every curry. I use a coffee grinder for small quantities of dry spices. A food processor can help to knead dough for bread, and it can also be used to chop or grate ingredients.
- A grater, a sieve, a rolling pin and board, a colander and a spice box to hold often-used spices are all invaluable.
- A pressure cooker, which every kitchen in India has for the everyday cooking of meats, lentils and desserts. Although not so fashionable in the West these days, it reduces cooking time and seals nutrients into the food.
- A *tava*, or flat griddle, or even a flat omelette pan, used for roasting breads such as roti.

Measures

I believe that every cook adds a special ingredient to his or her creation that makes it unique and distinct. This may be a little more or less of spices, herbs or main ingredients, or it could simply be the way in which everything is combined.

My recipes are for four people, and I encourage my readers to experiment with the amount of spices or herbs to suit individual tastes. If you wish to follow the recipes given, do stick to either the metric or the US/imperial measures. It is not a good idea to use a combination of both. The cup measures are equivalents for both metric and US/imperial measures.

Anyone who loves food and cooking knows that a cook's intuition with regard to measures and cooking times contributes immensely to the success and individuality of the final dish. Don't let the thought of this intimidate you – it's all simply a matter of practise. I hope that this book will inspire my readers to make the most of practical and accessible ayurvedic wisdom, coupled with good old common sense, to progress towards a lifestyle of good health and vitality.

MEASURE	METRIC	US/IMPERIAL
1 teaspoon	5 ml	1/6 fl oz
1 tablespoon	15 ml	1/2 fl oz
1 cup	250 ml	8 fl oz

GLOSSARY OF INGREDIENTS

All of these ingredients are readily available from Indian and Asian grocery stores, although you may be able to find some of them in your local shop.

asafoetida powder An extremely powerful-smelling spice used sparingly in Indian cooking. Asafoetida derives from the gum resin of particular species of giant fennel and helps to reduce gas in the stomach.

besan Fine flour made commercially by processing chickpeas (garbanzo beans). It is also known as chickpea flour.

black-eyed beans Small dried, cream-coloured beans with a black centre. Also known as black-eyed peas or cowpeas.

channa dal This dal, also known as Bengal gram, is made from chickpeas (garbanzo beans). The dried chickpeas are skinned and split, making the dal.

chickpeas These small legumes, also known as garbanzo beans, are a common feature in Indian cookery. They turn up in various forms, whether it be whole, skinned and split for dal or milled for flour. Chickpeas are usually sold dried and need to be soaked before cooking because of their tough skins.

dal Also spelled dhal, this is a spicy dish made with pulses and served with curries. The term 'dal' refers to any of the dried legumes, such as peas, mung beans and lentils, used in making the dish.

fenugreek leaves Also sold as methi, this popular Indian herb is used as either a vegetable or a flavouring. It is slightly bitter in taste. If you cannot buy fresh fenugreek leaves, the dried leaves are sold as kasuri methi in Indian grocery stores.

garam masala This literally means 'warming spices' and is a combination of spices used to aid digestion. The choices used can vary slightly, according to whether the garam masala is to be hot or fragrant.

ghee Highly prized in ayurveda because of its ability to aid absorption, ghee is simple enough to make your own (see page 124), or you can buy it commercially. Ghee is also used therapeutically in ayurveda. Also known as clarified butter.

jaggery Dehydrated sugarcane juice formed as a by-product during the manufacture of sugar. Sticky like molasses, jaggery has a distinctive musky flavour. You can substitute soft dark brown sugar (with a sizeable molasses content) at a pinch. Also known as gur in India.

khichadi A delicious stew made of mung beans, basmati rice, vegetables and spices (see page 97). A good meal at any time, it is also particularly useful when people are convalescing or a light, nutritious diet is required. Also known as kitchari or kitcheri.

masoor dal This dal is made from red lentils, which are skinned and split.

mung beans These are another type of dried bean found in wide use in Indian cookery. Unlike chickpeas, dried mung beans do not need to be soaked overnight before using and they cook much more quickly than chickpeas. They are sometimes sprouted for use in salads, and so on – an extremely simple process. Also known as green gram or golden gram, according to the colour of their skin.

mung dal This dal is made from dried mung beans. The mung beans are skinned and split, and the resulting split lentils are small, oval and yellow. Also known as moong dal.

tamarind A sour fruit with a distinctive tart flavour, tamarinds grow in pods. The pulp is sold in jars and can be diluted in a little water before use.

toor dal This dal is made from skinned and split yellow lentils, also called pigeon peas, which are sometimes available oiled. Also known as arhar dal.

urad dal The cream-coloured dal made from the skinned and split small black beans also known as black lentils. Also known as split black gram.

Soups & Starters

Deliciously fragrant soups or spicy little appetizers can set the tone and mood for the meal to follow, and they often provide a dash of dramatic colour as well. Although in India the entire meal is served as one event, without distinct courses, soups and starters are given on formal occasions. Clear soups and broths are easier to digest than creamy or thick ones, while rich soups are best in winter, when the contracting quality of colder weather helps to concentrate and strengthen agni, or digestive fire.

When you're selecting ingredients, bear in mind that, according to ayurvedic principles, it is best to eat foods when they are in season. If we respect nature and enjoy its offerings when we are meant to, we derive maximum benefit from its riches. Out-of-season foods are rarely as nutritious as naturally ripened or readied ones, so choose fresh ingredients that hint at the promise of the feast to follow.

Fragrant Carrot & Ginger Soup

This soup is a winter favourite in India, as its carotene content helps to protect against damage from pollution lingering in the heavy, cold air. Carrots contain vitamin A, which strengthens the eyes and ensures growth in children and adolescents. Oranges provide vitamin C, which helps to heal wounds and boosts resistance to infection. The vibrant orange colour of this soup creates an aura of warm energy to build immunity. This recipe will reduce vata and kapha, but people with a pitta constitution should limit the amount of ginger to a mere dash.

1 tablespoon sunflower oil

300 g (10 oz) juicy carrots, finely grated

2.5 cm (1 in) piece of cinnamon stick

½ teaspoon freshly grated ginger

100 ml (½ cup) freshly squeezed orange juice

½ teaspoon granulated sugar

½ teaspoon ground cumin

sea salt to taste

Preparation time: **10 minutes**
Cooking time: **25 minutes**
Serves: **4**

1 Heat the oil until hot in a heavy-bottomed saucepan. Then add the carrot, cinnamon and ginger, and stir for a few minutes. Pour in 600 ml (2 ½ cups) water. Bring to a boil, reduce the heat and simmer for about 15 minutes until the carrots are cooked through.

2 Allow the liquid to cool slightly, then blend or process until smooth. Add the orange juice, sugar, cumin and salt to taste.

3 Return the blended liquid to the pan and reheat.

4 Serve hot, with fresh crusty bread.

GAJAR
ADRAK
KA SHORBA

Red Onion Soup

It may seem logical to think that onions, being pungent, are warming, but in fact the opposite is true. Onions are cooling and therefore calm the body, while at the same time they inhibit digestion. The garlic in this recipe overcomes this, as it helps to stimulate agni. Cooking onions makes them light and sweet, and therefore balancing for pitta and vata. This is especially important for pitta, which is aggravated by raw onions. This pungency, however, is ideal for kapha. Red onions give this soup a zing of energy that boosts vitality and lifts the spirits.

1 tablespoon ghee

½ teaspoon cumin seed

2 large red onions, finely sliced

1 clove garlic, crushed

1 teaspoon barley flour

sea salt and freshly ground black pepper

1 tablespoon lemon juice

1 teaspoon freshly chopped coriander (cilantro) leaves

Preparation time: **10 minutes**
Cooking time: **25 minutes**
Serves: **4**

1 Heat the ghee in a heavy-bottomed pan and, when medium-hot, drop in the cumin seed.

2 As the seeds begin to darken, add the onion and fry until tender, about 10 minutes.

3 Add the garlic and stir through. Push the onion mixture to the sides of the pan, making a space in the middle, then reduce the heat. Sprinkle the flour into the ghee, and cook for a minute or so before stirring it into the onion mixture.

4 Add 600 ml (2 ½ cups) hot water and salt and pepper to taste. Bring to a boil.

5 Reduce the heat and simmer for 10 minutes. Remove from the heat, and add the lemon juice.

6 Serve warm, garnished with the coriander.

LAL PYAZ KA SHORBA

Spinach & Lentil Soup

We have all been raised to believe that eating spinach will make us strong. Spinach does contain a fair amount of iron, but it is also a source of potassium oxalate, which binds with calcium and makes the absorption of iron difficult. In ayurveda, spinach is considered cooling and soothing with light, dry qualities, and small amounts are good for all the doshas. The addition of lentils to this recipe provides a little heat to stimulate digestion. Green is a colour of balance, and this silky soup will help to relieve stress and emotional problems.

¼ teaspoon each freshly crushed ginger and garlic

1 tablespoon sunflower oil

1 medium onion, chopped

300 g (10 oz) fresh spinach, washed and drained

2 tablespoons yellow mung dal (split mung beans)

1 medium tomato, chopped

sea salt and freshly ground black pepper

1 bay leaf

single (light) cream, to serve (optional)

Preparation time: 10 minutes
Cooking time: 20 minutes
Serves: 4

1 Combine the crushed ginger and garlic to make a paste. Set aside.

2 Heat the oil in a heavy-bottomed pan until it is almost smoking, then add the onion. Sauté until tender, about 2–3 minutes.

3 Add the reserved ginger-garlic paste, and fry for a minute or so.

4 Roughly tear the spinach leaves and drop them into the pan, then add the mung dal and tomato. Stir through.

5 Pour in 600 ml (2 ½ cups) hot water, salt and pepper to taste and the bay leaf. Bring to a boil. Reduce the heat and simmer until done, about 15 minutes.

6 Remove from the heat, discard the bay leaf and blend or process the mixture to a puree.

7 Serve hot, swirled with cream if liked (but not for kapha types).

Lamb Broth Laced with Wheat Milk

Meat needs to be spiced in order to enhance agni. Here a host of spices join forces with ginger and garlic to make this delicious broth from the royal state of Hyderabad more digestible. In fact, it is often made for people who are convalescing to rebuild their strength. Although lamb is popular in Indian cookery, it is unsettling to all the doshas. The wheat milk in this recipe adds moistness, making the soup more balancing for vata and pitta. Kapha types are aggravated by significant amounts of both lamb and wheat, so should enjoy it only in small quantities.

150 g (5 oz) wheat flakes, soaked overnight in water

300 g (10 oz) neck of lamb, chopped

1 bay leaf

10 black peppercorns, crushed

3 whole cardamom pods, bruised

2 cloves, bruised

½ teaspoon each freshly crushed ginger and garlic, combined (see page 18)

3 teaspoons sunflower oil

1 medium onion, finely chopped

sea salt

pinch of saffron threads

Preparation time: 10 minutes
Cooking time: 1 hour plus overnight soaking
Serves: 4

1 Drain the soaked wheat and whizz in a blender with 150 ml (⅔ cup) fresh cold water. Squeeze out the thick wheat milk using a fine strainer. Set aside.

2 Put the lamb, bay leaf, peppercorns, cardamom, cloves and ginger-garlic paste in a deep, heavy saucepan with 600 ml (2½ cups) water. Bring to a boil, skimming off any scum that rises to the surface.

3 Cover the pan partially and simmer for about 40 minutes, or until the lamb is tender. Remove from the heat and strain the stock and reserve.

4 Lift the lamb onto a plate, and separate the flesh from the bones, reserving the meat and discarding the bones.

5 Heat the oil in a large saucepan and sauté the onion until golden. Pour in the lamb stock, season to taste with salt and add the reserved lamb.

6 Pour in the reserved wheat milk. Bring to a boil and remove from the heat.

7 Serve hot garnished with the saffron.

HALEEM
SHORBA

Chicken, Cumin & Potato Soup

Chicken, along with all other meats, carries red energy that boosts the circulation and provides vitality. Chicken and turkey are suitable for all the doshas and, wherever possible, should be chosen over red meat. Potatoes are sweet and astringent in taste and help to absorb excess water in the body without causing constipation or dryness. They are helpful to kapha and neutral to pitta, but aggravate vata types, who often find that they cause wind. If you have a vata constitution, substitute sweet potato for the potato, using only half the given quantity.

1 tablespoon sunflower oil

4 black peppercorns

1 bay leaf

1 teaspoon cumin seed

125 g (4 oz) boneless chicken, cubed

1 medium potato, peeled and diced

sea salt to taste

single (light) cream (optional)

Preparation time: **10 minutes**
Cooking time: **25 minutes**
Serves: **4**

1 Heat the oil in a deep saucepan until almost smoking, and add the peppercorns, bay leaf and cumin seed.

2 As the spices start to sizzle, add the chicken and stir for a minute or so.

3 Add the potato and salt, and pour in 600 ml (2 ½ cups) hot water. Bring to a boil, reduce the heat and simmer for 15 minutes.

4 Remove from the heat, and discard the bay leaf. Strain the soup, reserving the stock, and blend or process the chicken mixture with a little of the stock until very smooth.

5 Whisk the puree into the reserved stock, and adjust seasoning if necessary.

6 Serve hot, garnished with a swirl of cream if desired (but not for kapha types).

MURG

ALOO

KA SHORBA

Fresh Corn Fritters

Fresh cornbread is made every day in Punjab during the cold, misty winter. Grains of corn when roasted or made into flour are considered light and dry, making them ideal for kapha. Fresh corn is moist and provides better balance for pitta and vata.

The bright yellow energy of corn and the cleansing turmeric used in this recipe are said to stimulate the nervous system and will help you to be more alert and focused in your thinking.

2 cobs fresh sweetcorn, grated

2 tablespoons besan (chickpea flour)

½ teaspoon granulated sugar

¼ teaspoon ground turmeric

1 fresh green chilli, minced

¼ teaspoon each freshly crushed ginger and garlic, combined (see page 18)

1 tablespoon natural (plain) yoghurt

1 tablespoon freshly chopped coriander (cilantro) leaves

pinch of salt

sunflower oil, for deep-frying

Preparation time: **15 minutes**
Cooking time: **20 minutes**
Serves: **4**

1 Combine all the ingredients except the oil in a mixing bowl. Knead into a soft dough.

2 Heat the oil in a deep kadhai or wok over a high heat. Meanwhile, shape the dough into balls, or pakoras, about the size of a large cherry.

3 When the oil is hot, reduce the heat and gently drop in a few balls of dough. Fry until golden. Remove with a slotted spoon, drain on absorbent kitchen paper and set aside to keep warm.

4 Continue in this manner until all the balls have been fried. (You may need to adjust the heat as you cook so that the pakoras don't become too dark on the outside or remain uncooked in the centre.)

5 Serve warm with tomato ketchup for dipping and a salad of fresh greens.

Prawns Tossed in Green Herbs

Prawns and shrimp are excellent foods for vata, but if you're predominantly pitta or kapha, you had best enjoy them in moderation. They are, however, lower in saturated fats than most meats and therefore make a healthier option. Seafood is rich in iodine, which is essential for thyroid metabolism. A deficiency in this nutrient can also lower the body temperature.

The jewel green of this dish connects us to nature and helps to refresh and purify our systems. It also allows us to breathe slowly, deeply and healthily by relaxing our minds.

300 g (10 oz) large raw prawns (shrimp), peeled and deveined

3 tablespoons sunflower oil

lemon wedges (optional)

MARINADE

large bunch of fresh coriander (cilantro) leaves

large bunch of fresh mint leaves

½ teaspoon each freshly crushed ginger and garlic, combined (see page 18)

2 fresh green chillies, chopped

2 tablespoons freshly squeezed lemon juice

½ teaspoon garam masala

pinch of salt

Preparation time: **15 minutes**
Cooking time: **15 minutes**
Serves: **4**

1 Blend or process all the ingredients for the marinade until smooth, then marinate the prawns in the mixture for 10 minutes.

2 Heat the oil in a heavy-bottomed pan until almost smoking, and fry the prawns in batches until opaque and cooked.

3 Serve hot, garnished with lemon wedges, if liked.

Chicken in Spices & Honey

A chaat is a wonderful medley of meat, vegetables or fruits tossed in spices and herbs, and sprinkled with ginger. This one is sweetened with honey, which has dry properties and is therefore very good for kapha. Pitta types benefit from newly collected honey, the fresher the better, whereas vata types will find honey aggravating if they eat it too often. In colour therapy honey's yellow hue is representative of daylight and brings optimism.

300 g (10 oz) cooked chicken, cut into strips

1 medium onion, sliced

handful of fresh coriander (cilantro) leaves, chopped

lettuce leaves

½ teaspoon finely grated fresh ginger

HONEY DRESSING

¼ teaspoon roasted ground cumin*

¼ teaspoon chilli powder

a little rock salt

1 tablespoon sunflower oil

1 tablespoon honey

2 tablespoons lemon juice

Preparation time: **15 minutes**
Cooking time: **Nil**
Serves: **4**

1 Combine the ingredients for the dressing, mix thoroughly and set aside.

2 Gently mix the chicken, onion and coriander in a bowl. Pour the dressing over the top, and toss everything together.

3 Arrange a bed of lettuce on a serving plate and pile the chicken mixture on top. Serve with the ginger sprinkled over the top.

* If you cannot buy roasted ground cumin, simply dry-roast your own using ordinary ground cumin, in a small frying pan or skillet.

Spicy Chicken Wings

In this recipe ginger and garlic are the main flavourings, and these are excellent for vata because of their properties of dispelling gas. Both ginger and garlic are hot, and they help to stimulate the digestion and balance the heaviness of the chicken. Garlic contains all the tastes except sour and is used to treat respiratory problems. The red energy of this dish helps to activate the adrenal glands in order to build stamina.

300 g (10 oz) chicken wings, skin removed

sunflower oil for deep-frying

mint chutney, to serve (optional)

BATTER

125 g (1 cup) plain (all-purpose) flour

3/4 teaspoon each freshly crushed ginger and garlic, combined (see page 18)

1/2 teaspoon chilli powder

1/2 teaspoon garam masala

1/2 teaspoon ground turmeric

1/2 teaspoon baking powder

pinch of salt

Preparation time: **20 minutes**
Cooking time: **20 minutes**
Serves: **4**

1 Combine all the ingredients for the batter and gradually add enough water to make a thick consistency. Set aside.

2 Scrape the meat towards one end of each chicken wing and dip the wings in the batter.

3 Heat the oil in a deep frying pan (skillet) or kadhai. Lift each wing from the batter, and deep-fry in batches until crisp and golden, adjusting the heat as you go to ensure that the wings cook evenly but without becoming too brown. Drain on absorbent kitchen paper and keep warm.

4 Serve hot with with a prepared mint chutney, if liked.

MURG KI CHHARRIA

Baby Lentil Dumplings in Yoghurt

Yoghurt is considered a miracle food in India. It is well known for relieving the first churnings of an upset stomach, as well as nudging along a sluggish digestive system. It is ideal for vata, while kapha and pitta types could try yoghurt made from soya milk, which is less aggravating. Here the lentils are flavoured with a pinch of asafoetida, a strong, pungent spice that helps to prevent the formation of gas in the gut usually associated with legumes. In colour therapy yoghurt has a green ray, as it is derived from grass and thus is thought to be calming and peaceful.

300 ml (1¼ cups) natural (plain) yoghurt

1 teaspoon granulated sugar

a little rock salt

¼ teaspoon roasted ground cumin

handful of fresh coriander (cilantro) leaves, chopped

DUMPLING BATTER

150 g (5 oz) urad dal (split black lentils)

pinch of asafoetida powder

¼ teaspoon minced fresh green chilli

½ teaspoon freshly grated ginger

sunflower oil for deep-frying

Preparation time: 15 minutes plus 6 hours for soaking
Cooking time: 20 minutes
Serves: 4

1 First make the lentil dumpling batter. Soak the urad dal in cold water for 6 hours. Drain away the water, and blend or process the soaked gram to a fine paste.

2 Add the asafoetida, chilli and ginger to the paste, and mix well to make a thick batter.

3 Heat the oil until almost smoking in a deep frying pan or skillet, and drop in a tablespoon of the batter. Fry until crisp and golden. Remove the dumpling with a slotted spoon and immerse in a bowl of water. Lift out of the bowl and squeeze gently with your hands, then set aside. Adjust the heat to ensure even cooking and continue in the same manner with the rest of the batter.

4 Whisk the yoghurt with 4 tablespoons water, the sugar and rock salt in a separate bowl.

5 Place the fried dumplings in the seasoned yoghurt. Sprinkle the cumin over the top and garnish with the coriander.

6 Serve slightly chilled.

Seafood & Eggs

2

Ayurveda recognizes the warming qualities of fish and therefore recommends fish only for people with a predominantly vata constitution. Pitta types can enjoy other types of seafood such as prawns and shrimp, but people with a kapha constitution need to be careful with any offerings from the sea.

Fish is also a great source of minerals; however, the phosphorus present in most fish can upset reserves of bone-building calcium in our bodies. The addition of calcium-rich leafy greens to your meal will help to make it more balancing.

Contrary to popular belief, eggs are actually quite difficult to digest. People with a tendency towards high cholesterol should limit the number of eggs in their diet to two or three a week and check for a sluggish liver or chromium deficiency, which can sometimes lead to raised cholesterol levels.

Goan Fish Curry

The natural fat in the mackerel used in this recipe, along with the phosphorus, iodine and vitamins B and D, make it a complete, healthy food. Fish contains as much protein as meat and helps to build muscle. It is excellent for vata, good for pitta in moderation and tolerated by kapha in small amounts. Mackerel is associated with violet energy, which is both calming and stimulating. This recipe will help you to channel your energy in a creative manner.

4 dried red chillies, deseeded and soaked in a little water

1 small onion, roughly chopped

1 teaspoon ground coriander

2 teaspoons tamarind pulp soaked in a little water

1 teaspoon freshly minced garlic

sea salt

8 fillets of firm white fish such as cod, about 1 kg (2 lb)

1 tablespoon sunflower oil

300 ml (1¼ cups) coconut milk

Preparation time: **15 minutes**
Cooking time: **15 minutes**
Serves: **4**

1 Blend or process the chilli, onion, coriander, tamarind and garlic to a fine paste.

2 Season with salt to taste, and smear the paste over the fish. Reserve.

3 Heat the oil in a pan over a low heat and fry the marinated fish.

4 When the fish is nearly done, add the coconut milk and adjust the seasoning. Bring just to a boil, then remove from the heat immediately.

5 To reheat, gently warm the curry through – if coconut milk is boiled for too long, it separates.

6 Serve warm, with fluffy Boiled Rice (see page 96).

GOENCHI KODHI

Crab with Roasted Coconut

Coconut is sweet and cooling, and tones down the heating quality of the crab in this coastal Indian recipe. Kapha types have to be careful eating this, as both coconut and seafood aggravate this dosha. The crab, reputed to be an aphrodisiac, is considered to have a red energy (for passion and action) because it is an animal food, as well as a blue energy (many crabs have bluish shells). Both of these are balanced by the calming green energy of the coconut.

4 tablespoons sunflower oil

10 whole black peppercorns

6 cloves

2 teaspoons coriander seed

1 large onion, finely sliced

250 g (8 oz) freshly grated or desiccated (shredded) coconut

handful of fresh coriander (cilantro) leaves

3 fresh green chillies

½ tablespoon each freshly crushed ginger and garlic, combined (see page 18)

4 fresh crabs, about 250 g (8 oz) each, cleaned, claws retained and legs discarded

1 teaspoon ground turmeric

sea salt to taste

1 teaspoon freshly squeezed lemon juice

Preparation time: **15 minutes**
Cooking time: **40 minutes**
Serves: **4**

1 Heat 2 tablespoons of the oil in a deep, heavy frying pan or skillet until almost smoking. Add the peppercorns, cloves and coriander seed. Stir for a minute or so.

2 Add the onion and fry until brown – the colour of the dish depends on this step. Add the coconut and stir-fry until golden, taking care not to let the coconut mixture burn.

3 Cool the mixture slightly and blend or process to a paste with a few teaspoons of water. Reserve.

4 Blend or process the coriander leaves, chillies and ginger-garlic paste. Set aside.

5 Heat the remaining 2 tablespoons oil in a separate heavy-bottomed pan, and add the crabs. Fry until they turn red. Add the turmeric and salt.

6 Add the reserved green coriander paste, and fry for 5 minutes. Pour in the reserved coconut paste, and bring to a boil. Reduce the heat and simmer for about 10 minutes, or until the crabs are cooked. Remove from the heat, and stir in the lemon juice.

7 Serve hot, with Millet Bread (see page 103) and Green Beans with Corn (see page 71).

Mild Prawn & Coconut Curry

Prawns (shrimp) are considered quite heating in ayurveda, even when they are served cold in salads. They help to balance vata and can be tolerated by pitta as an occasional meal, but aggravate kapha. In this recipe, the prawns are cooled by the coconut milk, making the dish suitable for each of the doshas. People with a tendency towards high cholesterol should be wary of eating too much coconut. Indian women apply coconut oil to their hair to keep it glossy and thick. Its green energy helps to promote feelings of rejuvenation.

3 tablespoons sunflower oil

5 fresh or dried curry leaves

1 teaspoon freshly crushed garlic

500 g (1 lb) large prawns (shrimp), peeled and deveined

1 teaspoon chilli powder

1 teaspoon garam masala

1 tablespoon tomato puree (paste)

sea salt

300 ml (1¼ cups) coconut milk*

handful of coriander (cilantro) leaves, freshly chopped

Preparation time: **15 minutes**
Cooking time: **20 minutes**
Serves: **4**

1 Heat the oil until almost smoking in a heavy-bottomed frying pan or skillet, and fry the curry leaves and garlic for a minute.

2 Add the prawns, chilli powder and garam masala, and stir-fry over a low heat for 5 minutes.

3 Next add the tomato puree, salt to taste and a few tablespoons of hot water, and simmer until the prawns are cooked, about 7 minutes.

4 Pour in the coconut milk, bring to a boil and remove the pan from the heat.

5 Garnish with the coriander, and serve with Dried Fruit Pulao (see page 99).

* The coconut milk in this recipe cannot be replaced with cow's milk.

JHINGA
MALAI KADHI

Sindhi-style Eggs

In Sindhi 'seyal' means to cook with onions and herbs. This recipe is flavoured with coriander (cilantro), which is excellent for all the doshas. Fresh coriander cools a meal, and this may be the reason why it is the favoured garnish for so many hot, spicy Indian curries. Its green energy tones the heart and helps to lower blood pressure. Eggs are hot, heavy and oily. They are also fairly difficult to digest, so don't overdo them in your diet.

3 tablespoons sunflower oil

2 large onions, grated and squeezed (reserve juice)

½ tablespoon each freshly crushed ginger and garlic, combined (see page 18)

1 teaspoon ground cumin

1 teaspoon garam masala

½ teaspoon ground turmeric

½ teaspoon chilli powder

½ teaspoon ground mace

3 medium tomatoes, chopped

150 ml (²/₃ cup) natural (plain) yoghurt, beaten

150 g (5 oz) fresh coriander (cilantro), finely chopped

8 hard-boiled eggs, peeled and halved

Preparation time: **15 minutes**
Cooking time: **20 minutes**
Serves: **4**

1 Heat the oil until almost smoking in a heavy-bottomed pan, and fry the onions until translucent. Add the ginger–garlic paste, and fry for another minute or so.

2 Add the cumin, garam masala, turmeric, chilli powder and mace, then stir before adding the tomato. Cook until the tomato is mushy, then pour in the reserved onion juice.

3 Stir in the yoghurt and coriander, and simmer for 5 minutes over a low heat.

4 Arrange the halved eggs in a serving dish and pour the curry over the top. Serve hot, with Flatbread (see page 100) and Potato & Yoghurt Salad (see page 111).

SEYAL

ANDE

Egg Croquettes

Egg whites possess cool, light properties when eaten on their own, and this makes them an excellent source of protein for pitta and kapha. Vata is calmed when eggs are cooked well. This tasty accompaniment derives its crispness from the rice flour used in the batter. This fine, white flour calms pitta and vata, and, in small quantities, is good for kapha. Rice contains yellow energy, which helps to purify the blood.

sunflower oil for deep-frying

8 large hard-boiled eggs, peeled and halved

Preparation time: 10 minutes
Cooking time: 20 minutes
Serves: 4

BATTER

2 tablespoons besan (chickpea flour)

2 tablespoons rice flour

¼ teaspoon chilli powder

¼ teaspoon ground turmeric

¼ teaspoon ground coriander

pinch of baking powder

pinch of salt

1 Combine the ingredients for the batter, and stir in enough cold water to make a batter of dropping consistency.

2 Heat the oil until almost smoking in a deep-sided frying pan or deep-fryer. Dip each egg half in the batter, shake off any excess and deep-fry until a rich golden colour.

3 Drain on absorbent kitchen paper. Continue in this way until all the egg halves have been cooked.

4 Serve hot, with agni-igniting tomato ketchup and a green salad.

MUTTAI BAJJI

Egg & Pineapple Curry

Although eggs are not easily digestible, when combined with cooling pineapple they become more balanced. Sweet pineapples are considered tridoshic, i.e. they can be tolerated by all the doshas. They can aggravate kapha, however, if eaten in excess. The yellow colour of pineapple is especially associated with the liver, strengthening it and ensuring good digestion. A blockage or a reduction in the functioning of the liver often manifests itself as 'yellow', as seen in jaundice or hepatitis, for instance.

4 tablespoons sunflower oil

1 large onion, sliced

½ tablespoon each freshly crushed ginger and garlic, combined (see page 18)

1 teaspoon poppy seed

2 fresh green chillies, chopped

handful of fresh mint leaves

½ teaspoon cumin seed

1 teaspoon ground turmeric

1 teaspoon garam masala

2 tomatoes, chopped

8 hard-boiled eggs, peeled and halved

sea salt

300 ml (1¼ cups) coconut milk

2 large rings fresh pineapple, chopped

pinch of saffron threads

Preparation time: **15 minutes**
Cooking time: **25 minutes**
Serves: **4**

1 Heat 2 tablespoons of the oil, and fry the onion for 5 minutes until soft. Add the ginger-garlic paste, poppy seed and chilli. Stir-fry for another minute or so.

2 Remove from the heat, cool slightly and blend or process to a paste with the mint leaves. Set aside.

3 Heat the remaining 2 tablespoons oil until almost smoking in a heavy-bottomed pan, and add the cumin seed. When the seeds begin to crackle, add the turmeric, garam masala and tomato. Stir until the tomato is mushy.

4 Add the reserved onion paste, eggs and salt to taste. Pour in the coconut milk, and bring to a boil.

5 Reduce the heat and simmer for a minute before removing from the heat and adding the pineapple and saffron.

6 Serve hot, with Boiled Rice (see page 96) and Mixed Peppers with Cashews (see page 75).

Spicy Scrambled Eggs with Mushrooms

Mushrooms are light and dry, and are a suitable food for pitta and kapha. When spiced, as they are here, they are also beneficial to vata. In ayurveda, however, mushrooms are considered to be 'tamasic', i.e. they belong to a group of foods felt to promote lethargy and make the brain sluggish. They also increase ama, so it is suggested that you eat them in moderation. In this wonderful recipe they counteract the heavy oiliness of the eggs. In colour therapy eggs are full of go-getting red energy, while mushrooms have an indigo ray that is soporific.

1 tablespoon sunflower oil

½ teaspoon cumin seed

1 fresh green chilli, minced

½ teaspoon ground turmeric

150 g (5 oz) mushrooms, sliced

8 large eggs, beaten and seasoned with

sea salt and freshly ground black pepper

2 tablespoons chopped fresh coriander (cilantro) leaves

Preparation time: 10 minutes
Cooking time: 10 minutes
Serves: 4

1 Heat the oil until almost smoking in a heavy-bottomed frying pan or skillet, and add the cumin seed. When the seeds begin to sizzle and darken, add the chilli. Fry for a few seconds.

2 Sprinkle in the turmeric and stir through, then add the mushrooms. Stir for a few minutes until they begin to soften.

3 Pour in the egg and stir quickly to scramble – this is important to prevent the egg becoming rubbery and watery. Remove the pan from the heat before the egg has cooked completely. Add the coriander, and allow the egg to finish cooking in the pan.

4 Serve hot with Flatbread (see page 100), Garlic-flavoured Lentils (see page 89) and a deliciously crisp, leafy salad to add a sweep of green energy.

ANDE
AUR KHUMB
KI BHURJI

Eggs with Spicy Lemon Okra

Okra is a marvellously healthy vegetable if you don't mind its sticky, slippery feel. Its sliminess (known as slakshna in ayurveda) helps lubrication and hence digestion. As a bonus, it is also rich in calcium and vitamins B1 and B2. It is fairly well tolerated by all the doshas and is considered soothing and diuretic. Eggs are a good source of protein, but people with a tendency towards high cholesterol would do well to limit them to a couple a week. The glowing green energy of okra also helps to increase immunity to illness and infection.

450 g (1 lb) fresh okra, washed and drained well

3 tablespoons sunflower oil

½ teaspoon fenugreek seed

pinch of asafoetida powder

½ teaspoon ground turmeric

½ teaspoon chilli powder

½ teaspoon ground coriander

sea salt

1 tablespoon freshly squeezed lemon juice

4 large eggs

freshly ground black pepper

Preparation time: **15 minutes**
Cooking time: **25 minutes**
Serves: **4**

1 Make sure that the okra is completely dry before you use it, as any extra moisture will make it too slimy. Slice each okra down the middle, discarding the top.

2 Heat 2 tablespoons of the oil until almost smoking in a heavy-bottomed frying pan or skillet, and add the fenugreek seed.

3 When the seeds turn brown, add the asafoetida, turmeric, chilli powder and coriander.

4 Stir, and add the sliced okra. Season with salt to taste, and mix well. Sprinkle lemon juice over the top – the acid in the lemon helps to keep the sliminess within the okra. Cook uncovered, stirring occasionally to prevent sticking, for 15 minutes, or until done. Remove from the heat, and spoon into a warmed serving bowl.

5 Heat the remaining 1 tablespoon oil in a skillet, and gently break the eggs into it, keeping the yolks intact. Cover and cook for a minute. Gently lift out the eggs, drain and place over the okra.

6 Season with salt and pepper, and serve. Enjoy with Whole Red Lentils with Onion & Yoghurt (see page 86) and Flatbread (see page 100).

Southern Fried Fish

This South Indian delicacy is flavoured with curry leaves, a herb that grows easily in many Indian homes. Curry leaves, like bay leaves, are usually removed from the food before it is eaten. However, they are not as tough as bay leaves and, if you can bear a little bitterness, chewing them almost guarantees good health. Buy curry leaves fresh if possible, as the dried ones simply do not have the same potency. They are excellent for kapha and pitta, and are used in ayurveda as a tonic, carminative and digestive.

8 cod or any other firm white fish fillets, about 1 kg (2 lb)

4 tablespoons sunflower oil

1 teaspoon mustard seed

10 curry leaves

1 small onion, chopped

wedges of lime to garnish

2 tablespoons freshly chopped coriander (cilantro) leaves

MARINADE

a little sea salt

1 teaspoon freshly crushed garlic

½ teaspoon cracked black pepper

1 teaspoon chilli powder

1 teaspoon ground coriander

1 teaspoon ground turmeric

Preparation time: 10 minutes plus 30 minutes for marinating
Cooking time: 20 minutes
Serves: 4

1 Combine all the marinade ingredients and mix to a paste. Smear over the fish and leave to marinate in the refrigerator for 30 minutes.

2 Heat the oil until almost smoking in a shallow frying pan or skillet, and add the mustard seed. As the seeds being to crackle, add the curry leaves. Fry for a minute or so.

3 Add the onion and allow to soften for 5-7 minutes, until translucent and golden. Gently place the fish in the oil and fry over a low heat, turning occasionally until done, about 10 minutes.

4 Serve hot with the lime wedges and a sprinkling of chopped coriander. This dish is especially good when accompanied by Boiled Rice (see page 96) and Coriander Dal (see page 88).

MEEN VARUVAL

Pan-fried Fish with Spinach

This recipe comes from the northwest of India and is a good example of how foods can be combined for healthy results. Fish is a great source of vitamins B and D (essential for the absorption of calcium) and minerals, but the phosphorus in most fish can deplete our stores of calcium. Some fish, such as tuna or sardines, are rich in calcium, but adding calcium-rich foods such as leafy greens to your meal will also balance your calcium intake. According to colour therapy, the green of spinach helps to lower blood pressure and soothe the nerves.

8 pieces of cod or any firm white fish, about 1 kg (2 lb)

½ teaspoon ground turmeric

sea salt

4 tablespoons sunflower oil

1 large onion, sliced

½ tablespoon each freshly crushed ginger and garlic, combined (see page 18)

2 medium tomatoes, chopped

300 g (10 oz) fresh spinach, lightly boiled or steamed, then drained well

1 teaspoon dried fenugreek leaves (sold as kasuri methi in Indian grocery stores)

1 teaspoon garam masala

½ teaspoon fresh ginger strips

Preparation time: 15 minutes
Cooking time: 25 minutes
Serves: 4

1 Smear the fish with the turmeric and a little salt. Marinate in the refrigerator for 30 minutes.

2 Heat the oil until almost smoking in a heavy-bottomed pan, and fry the marinated fish for about 8 minutes, taking care not to break it. Drain the fish on absorbent kitchen paper and set aside.

3 Add the onion and fry until soft. Add the ginger-garlic paste and tomato. Stir until mushy.

4 Add the spinach, fenugreek leaves, garam masala and salt to taste. Cook for 5–7 minutes.

5 To serve, place the fish on a warm serving platter and top with the spinach mixture. Sprinkle the ginger strips on top. Serve accompanied by Flatbread (see page 100).

MACCHI PALAK

Chicken & Lamb

In early times, long before the advent of modern agricultural methods, when animals were found only in their natural habitat, their flesh was considered nourishing. Today's meat is often highly processed and produced under artificial conditions, so it does not meet the exacting standards of ayurvedic nutrition. If you do eat meat and poultry, it is essential that you combine it with fruits, vegetables and legumes, preferably organic, which aid digestion and create power in the body. Lamb, in particular, needs to be lightened to make it healthy as it is not well tolerated by any of the doshas – although it has become very popular in India and is a now a regular feature of the diet. All the doshas should eat it only in moderation. Also, mixing meat with dairy products generally reduces its digestibility, although yoghurt is an exception to this as it helps absorption in the digestive tract. As a general rule, vata can tolerate beef, chicken and duck, while kapha and pitta are most suited to rabbit and chicken.

Goan Chicken with Coriander

In ayurveda green is seen as nature's colour and is considered refreshing and restorative. It works on our emotions to free us of stress and strain. Green chillies contain more vitamin C (helpful in boosting overall immunity) per gram than many oranges. Here green chillies are combined with high-protein chicken, which helps to build and maintain the muscles. Chicken in itself is warming and heavy to digest.

8 large chicken drumsticks

3 tablespoons freshly squeezed lemon juice

5 tablespoons sunflower oil

sea salt

MARINADE

300 g (10 oz) fresh coriander (cilantro) leaves

3 fresh green chillies

2 teaspoons each freshly crushed ginger and garlic

¼ teaspoon cumin seed

¼ teaspoon ground turmeric

½ teaspoon garam masala

½ teaspoon granulated sugar

Preparation time: 1 hour
Cooking time: 40 minutes
Serves: 4

1 Lightly pierce the chicken legs with a skewer. Sprinkle them with the lemon juice, 2 tablespoons of the oil and salt. Set aside.

2 Blend or process the coriander, chilli, ginger, garlic, cumin, turmeric, garam masala and sugar until smooth and velvety. Smear the chicken with the coriander paste and marinate, covered, in the refrigerator for 30 minutes.

3 Place the chicken legs on a baking tray or sheet, and drizzle with the remaining 3 tablespoons oil. Cook under a medium-hot grill (broiler), turning and basting frequently, until tender and the juices from the meatiest part of the drumstick run clear when tested with a skewer.

4 Serve hot, with a mildly flavoured rice (try adding a pinch of turmeric to the rice while cooking it) and a crisp green salad.

MURG CAFREAL

Chicken Curry with Fennel

The principal flavourings in this South Indian dish are cool and bitter curry leaves and sweet and cooling fennel seeds. Ayurveda uses curry leaves as a stimulant, and eating a few every morning is said to help to dispel wastes from the body. Pitta types especially benefit from fennel. A combination of fennel, ground cumin and coriander seed is one of India's most respected tonics to improve and stimulate agni.

3 tablespoons sunflower oil

2.5-cm (1-in) piece of cinnamon stick

1 teaspoon fennel seed

15 curry leaves

1 large onion, chopped

½ tablespoon each freshly crushed ginger and garlic, combined (see page 18)

½ teaspoon ground turmeric

½ teaspoon chilli powder

½ teaspoon ground coriander

2 tomatoes, chopped

600 g (1¼ lb) boneless chicken, cubed

sea salt

300 ml (1¼ cups) coconut milk

1 teaspoon tamarind pulp, diluted in a little water

Preparation time: **15 minutes**
Cooking time: **30 minutes**
Serves: **4**

1 Heat the oil until almost smoking in a heavy-bottomed pan, and add the cinnamon and fennel seed. When the seeds have started to sizzle, add the curry leaves.

2 Add the onion and sauté until golden, about 7 minutes, then add the ginger–garlic paste, turmeric, chilli powder and coriander. Stir for a couple of minutes.

3 Add the tomato and cook until soft.

4 Next add the chicken and salt to taste, and cook until nearly done, about 15 minutes.

5 Pour in the coconut milk, bring to a boil, then reduce the heat and continue cooking for a further 5 minutes or so.

6 Add the tamarind juice, simmer for a minute and remove from the heat.

7 Serve hot, with steamed rice.

Bengali-style Chicken with Sweet Yoghurt

Traditionally, a special yoghurt set with raw cane sugar is used in this recipe. I have substituted honey-flavoured yoghurt for this; it works just as well and adds a rich sweetness. Also, as yoghurt is too sour for pitta and too moist for kapha, the sweet, drying qualities of honey balance it, making the dish more suitable for both of these doshas. The raisins act as a gentle laxative and, along with the deep yellow colour of this dish, help in clearing the system.

1 large onion, chopped

½ tablespoon each freshly crushed ginger and garlic, combined (see page 18)

2 tablespoons raw cashew nuts

1 teaspoon almonds

1 tablespoon raisins

600 g (1¼ lb) chicken legs, skinned

300 ml (1¼ cups) thick Greek-style yoghurt with honey

a little sea salt

3 tablespoons sunflower oil

2 bay leaves

4 green cardamom pods, bruised

½ teaspoon garam masala

½ teaspoon ground turmeric

Preparation time: **15 minutes**
Cooking time: **40 minutes**
Serves: **4**

1 Coarsely blend or process the onion and ginger-garlic paste. Process the cashews, almonds and raisins separately, and set this mixture aside.

2 Smear the chicken with the onion mixture, yoghurt and salt.

3 Heat the oil until almost smoking in a heavy-bottomed pan, and drop in the bay leaves and cardamom. Add the chicken, garam masala and turmeric. Pour in about 125 ml (½ cup) hot water.

4 Bring to a boil, reduce the heat and simmer until the chicken is tender, about 30 minutes. Stir in the nut-raisin mixture, simmer for another minute and remove from the heat.

5 Serve hot with Cornbread (see page 104), which will enhance the bright, happy qualities of yellow associated with this meal.

Kashmiri Chicken with Cardamom

This simple yet festive recipe highlights the use of cardamom in North Indian cookery. Cardamom is a highly fragrant spice and has been used for centuries as a digestive cure for stomach disorders and heartburn. It is also simmered in milk and honey to help reverse impotency. Two main varieties of cardamom are used in Indian cooking, namely green and black. Each has different properties. The green cardamom in this recipe lightens the heaviness of the meat, making it easier to digest. The earthy colours of the dish remind us of the grounding qualities of nature.

4 tablespoons sunflower oil

3 medium onions, sliced

600 g (1¼ lb) chicken breast, skinned and diced

300 ml (1¼ cups) natural (plain) yoghurt

sea salt

150 g (5 oz) fresh coriander (cilantro) leaves, chopped

10 green cardamom pods, crushed

Preparation time: **10 minutes**
Cooking time: **30 minutes**
Serves: **4**

1 Heat 2 tablespoons of the oil until almost smoking in a heavy-bottomed pan, and fry the onions until golden. Remove with a slotted spoon, and blend or process to a paste.

2 Heat the remaining 2 tablespoons oil in the same pan. Add the onion paste and chicken, and mix well. Cook for about 10 minutes over a medium heat.

3 Pour in the yoghurt and 150 ml (⅔ cup) water, and season to taste with salt. Bring to a boil, reduce the heat and simmer until the chicken is cooked, about 15 minutes.

4 Add the coriander and cardamom, simmer for another minute and remove from the heat.

5 Serve hot, with Flatbread (see page 100).

DHANIVAL KORMA

Chicken with Fenugreek

In India, fenugreek seeds in sugared balls mixed with dried fruits are given to new mothers to promote lactation and natural weight loss. The leaves are sold fresh or dried (the latter are available as kasuri methi in Indian grocery stores) and are said to activate blood and hair cell development and to relieve a chronic cough. The rich green colour, too, helps to balance acid and alkali levels in the body.

4 tablespoons sunflower oil

1 teaspoon each freshly crushed ginger and garlic, combined (see page 18)

2 large onions, grated

600 g (1¼ lb) boneless chicken, cubed

¼ teaspoon chilli powder

¼ teaspoon ground turmeric

1 teaspoon garam masala

sea salt

3 tablespoons concentrated tomato puree (paste)

125 g (4 oz) dried fenugreek leaves (kasuri methi), soaked in a little water

Preparation time: **10 minutes**
Cooking time: **25 minutes**
Serves: 4

1 Heat the oil until almost smoking in a heavy-bottomed pan, and lightly fry the ginger-garlic paste. Squeeze the onion, reserve the juice and add to the pan. Stir until golden.

2 Add the chicken, chilli powder, turmeric, garam masala and salt. Mix well.

3 Next add the tomato puree, reserved onion juice and just enough hot water to make a thick curry.

4 Tip in the fenugreek leaves with their soaking water. Reduce the heat and cook until the chicken is done, about 20 minutes.

5 Serve hot, with Flatbread (see page 100).

MURG METHI

Chicken in Whole Spices

This simple North Indian dish needs hardly any preparation, and the whole spices used make it wonderfully aromatic. One of the prime spices here is cinnamon, which keeps the stomach strong and working effectively. It is helpful in reducing kapha and is therefore found in many cough mixtures. Similarly, cloves are bitingly sharp and pungent, and are a great digestive aid. Caraway seeds are beneficial to vata and kapha, and can be handled by pitta in moderation. The orange ray of cumin and ginger in this dish acts as a tonic and stimulates the body and mind.

4 tablespoons sunflower oil

2 bay leaves

4 cardamom pods

2.5-cm (1-in) piece of cinnamon stick

½ teaspoon caraway seed

7 cloves

2 dried red chillies

600 g (1¼ lb) chicken breast, skinned and diced

8 cloves garlic

1 teaspoon sliced fresh ginger

150 g (5 oz) baby onions, peeled

2 tablespoons chopped coriander (cilantro) leaves

2 tablespoons chopped fresh mint leaves

½ teaspoon ground turmeric

sea salt

300 ml (1¼ cups) natural (plain) yoghurt, beaten

Preparation time: **15 minutes**
Cooking time: **30 minutes**
Serves: **4**

1 Heat the oil until almost smoking in a heavy-bottomed pan, and add the bay leaves, cardamom, cinnamon, caraway seed, cloves and chillies.

2 When the spices start to sizzle, add the chicken and sauté for about 7 minutes, stirring occasionally.

3 Add the remaining ingredients except the yoghurt, and stir well. Add 150 ml (⅔ cup) hot water and bring to a boil. Reduce the heat, and cook until the chicken is nearly done, about 15 minutes.

4 Next add the yoghurt, heat through and remove from the heat.

5 Serve hot, with Millet Bread (see page 103) or Flatbread (see page 100).

Chicken with Tomatoes & Sweetcorn

This tangy dish derives its flavour from the tomatoes that make its sauce. Ripe, red tomatoes are very rich in both vitamins A and C, useful for growth and strong muscles. However, they are warm in potency, and too many tomatoes only aggravate pitta. Kapha types should avoid eating them too often. Their vibrant red colour will help to boost circulation when you are cold or tired.

4 tablespoons sunflower oil

1 teaspoon each freshly crushed ginger and garlic, combined (see page 18)

2 medium onions, finely chopped

600 g (1¼ lb) chicken legs, skinned

150 g (5 oz) cooked sweetcorn kernels

½ teaspoon chilli powder

1 teaspoon garam masala

1 bay leaf

250 g (8 oz) ripe red tomatoes, chopped

2 tablespoons concentrated tomato puree (paste)

sea salt

1 large green pepper, deseeded and diced

handful of fresh coriander (cilantro) leaves, chopped

Preparation time: 15 minutes
Cooking time: 40 minutes
Serves: 4

1 Heat the oil until almost smoking in a heavy-bottomed pan, and fry the ginger-garlic paste for a minute. Add the onion and fry until golden.

2 Add the chicken and stir-fry for 10 minutes.

3 Next add all the ingredients except the green pepper and coriander to the pan, and cook until the chicken is tender, about 15 minutes. You may need to add a little water to prevent the curry becoming too dry.

4 Add the green pepper, simmer for a minute and remove from the heat.

5 Garnish with the coriander and serve hot, with fresh crusty bread.

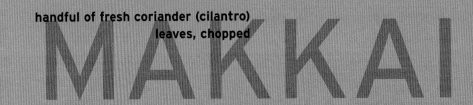
MURG MAKKAI

Spicy Chicken Drumsticks

The curative properties of garlic in relation to asthma and lung conditions are well known. It purifies the blood and keeps the skin glowing. Frying garlic lightly enhances its therapeutic action. Being hot and pungent, it is especially good for vata and kapha, but aggravates pitta. The golden-brown colour of this dish signifies optimism and will dispel gloom.

600 g (1¼ lb) chicken drumsticks, skinned

sunflower oil for basting

sliced onion and lemon wedges, to garnish (optional)

MARINADE

1 teaspoon freshly crushed garlic

½ teaspoon freshly crushed ginger

1 teaspoon freshly minced green chilli

1 teaspoon freshly chopped coriander (cilantro) leaves

1 teaspoon garam masala

2 tablespoons freshly squeezed lemon juice

sea salt

Preparation time: 15 minutes plus 2 hours for marinating
Cooking time: 45 minutes
Serves: 4

1 Make gashes in the chicken and set aside.

2 Combine all the ingredients for the marinade in a glass or ceramic dish, and add the chicken. Marinate in the refrigerator for a couple of hours.

3 Preheat the oven to 200°C (400°F, gas mark 6).

4 Arrange the marinated drumsticks on a greased baking tray or pan, drizzle with oil and bake for about 45 minutes, basting the chicken often with the cooking juices.

5 Serve hot, garnished with onion slices and wedges of lemon, if desired.

KALMI

KABAB

Chicken in Pickling Spices

The long list of ingredients in this energizing recipe should not deter you from making it. Fenugreek seeds are good for diabetics, peppercorns are stimulating, aniseed aids the digestion and mustard seeds are antiseptic. This chicken dish will benefit both vata and kapha, but pitta may find it too fiery (although a small amount should not do any harm). The warm brown colour is considered uplifting to the spirit.

4 tablespoons sunflower oil

1 tablespoon each freshly crushed ginger and garlic, combined (see page 18)

2 medium onions, sliced

600 g (1¼ lb) boneless chicken, cubed

sea salt

3 dried red chillies, deseeded

1 teaspoon mustard seed

10 black peppercorns

½ teaspoon fenugreek seed

1 teaspoon aniseed

½ teaspoon asafoetida powder

1 bay leaf

½ teaspoon ground turmeric

½ teaspoon chilli powder

1 teaspoon garam masala

150 ml (⅔ cup) natural (plain) yoghurt

Preparation time: **15 minutes**
Cooking time: **25 minutes**
Serves: **4**

1 Heat 2 tablespoons of the oil until almost smoking in a heavy-bottomed pan. Add the ginger-garlic paste and fry for a couple of minutes before adding the onion. Fry for another 7 minutes or so, until the onion is brown and crisp.

2 Add the chicken and salt to taste, and cook for a further 5 minutes. Add 150 ml (⅔ cup) hot water, and cook over a low heat until the chicken is nearly done, about 8 minutes.

3 Heat the remaining 2 tablespoons oil in a deep-sided frying pan or skillet, and add the chillies, mustard seed, peppercorns, fenugreek seed, aniseed and asafoetida. When the spices start to sizzle and sputter, add the bay leaf, turmeric, chilli powder and garam masala.

4 Beat the yoghurt slightly and stir in immediately. Pour the yoghurt mixture into the chicken, and cook for 5 more minutes to heat through, without bringing to a boil.

5 Serve hot, with Flatbread (see page 100).

Spicy Chicken with Green Peas

This soothing recipe combines the colour qualities of the red from the meat and the green from the peas to promote balance and harmony. Green peas are astringent in taste and as a result are considered healing. They help to absorb moisture and fat, and can assist a weight-loss programme. On the other hand, however, eating green peas to excess can lead to constipation. As they are gas-promoting, they aggravate vata, but they can be handled well by people of both pitta and kapha constitutions.

3 tablespoons sunflower oil

1 teaspoon each freshly crushed ginger and garlic, combined (see page 18)

2 medium onions, coarsely grated

500 g (1 lb) lean chicken mince (ground chicken)

½ teaspoon ground turmeric

½ teaspoon chilli powder

1 teaspoon garam masala

sea salt

2 medium tomatoes, chopped

150 g (5 oz) fresh or frozen green peas

freshly chopped coriander (cilantro) leaves, to garnish (optional)

Preparation time: **10 minutes**
Cooking time: **30 minutes**
Serves: **4**

1 Heat the oil until almost smoking in a heavy-bottomed pan, and fry the ginger–garlic paste for a minute or so.

2 Add the onion and fry until juice has evaporated and the onion starts to turn golden.

3 Next add the chicken and stir for a couple of minutes. Tip in the turmeric, chilli powder, garam masala and salt to taste. Cook for 5 minutes, stirring frequently.

4 Add the tomato and peas, and pour in 150 ml (⅔ cup) hot water. Bring to a boil. Reduce the heat and simmer until cooked, about 20 minutes.

5 Serve sprinkled with coriander if wished and accompanied by a soft bread of your choice.

Crispy Marinated Lamb Chops

This high-protein recipe is especially good for people who have a very physical occupation or do any form of vigorous exercise. The heaviness of the meat is countered by a whole host of spices, including cumin, which is an excellent aid to digestion. It helps to remove toxins from the body and tones the digestive tract. Cumin's orange ray also strengthens the immune system, making us resistant to ills brought on by overwork or fatigue.

3 tablespoons sunflower oil, plus extra for deep-frying

5 fresh red chillies

½ teaspoon fennel seed

1 teaspoon cumin seed

5 black peppercorns

½ tablespoon each freshly crushed ginger and garlic, combined (see page 18)

1 medium onion, sliced

1 teaspoon garam masala

½ teaspoon ground turmeric

sea salt

600 g (1¼ lb) lamb loin chops

2 fresh medium eggs, beaten

1 tablespoon freshly chopped coriander (cilantro) leaves

3 tablespoons wholemeal (whole-wheat) flour

lemon wedges, to garnish (optional)

Preparation time: **15 minutes**
Cooking time: **45 minutes**
Serves: **4**

1 Heat the 3 tablespoons sunflower oil until almost smoking in a frying pan or skillet, and add the chillies, fennel seed, cumin seed and peppercorns.

2 As the spices start to crackle, add the ginger–garlic paste. Stir and add the onion. Fry until golden. Add the garam masala, turmeric and salt to taste. Mix well.

3 Remove from the heat, cool slightly and blend or process to a puree.

4 Coat the lamb chops in the onion mixture, and set aside.

5 Combine the eggs, coriander and flour in a mixing bowl.

6 Heat the extra oil in a deep frying pan. Dip a few chops in the egg batter and gently lower into the oil. Fry in batches for 7-8 minutes until done. Adjust the heat to ensure even cooking. Drain the chops on absorbent kitchen paper and keep warm. Continue until all the chops are fried.

7 Serve at once, with wedges of lemon, if desired, and a Lettuce, Grape & Mango Salad (see page 115).

Southern Ginger Lamb

Ginger is an excellent digestive and is considered hot, pungent and stimulating. The fresh root is usually used, which is good for vata, but fine, dried powder can be substituted for kapha. Both fresh and dried ginger work wonders in stimulating the appetite. Fresh ginger juice is traditionally mixed with honey to relieve coughs and colds, and the orange energy of ginger assists the functioning of the circulatory system.

3 tablespoons freshly crushed ginger

1 teaspoon chilli powder

1 teaspoon ground coriander

1 teaspoon ground turmeric

sea salt

600 g (1¼ lb) lean boneless lamb, cubed

3 tablespoons sunflower oil

2.5-cm (1-in) piece of cinnamon stick

4 green cardamom pods, crushed

4 cloves

2 medium onions, chopped

1 teaspoon freshly minced garlic

300 ml (1¼ cups) coconut milk

Preparation time: 10 minutes plus 2 hours for marinating
Cooking time: 45 minutes
Serves: 4

1 Combine the ginger, chilli powder, coriander, turmeric and salt to taste in a glass or ceramic dish. Add the lamb, and marinate in the refrigerator for a couple of hours.

2 Heat the oil until almost smoking in a heavy-bottomed pan, and fry the cinnamon, cardamom and cloves. Add the onion and stir until golden.

3 Tip in the minced garlic and fry for another minute, then add the marinated lamb and stir-fry for 10 minutes. Adjust the seasoning, pour in 300 ml (1¼ cups) hot water and bring to a boil. Reduce the heat and simmer until the lamb is cooked, about 35 minutes.

4 Pour in the coconut milk and heat through, but do not allow to boil. Remove from the heat.

5 Serve with Dried Fruit Pulao (see page 99) or Boiled Rice (see page 96).

INJI KARI
KOZHAMBU

Bamboo-skewered Lamb Curry

In this recipe cloves join forces with other garam masala, or hot, spices to provide heat and fragrance. Although cloves are quite heating - you can feel your tongue smarting if you bite into them - they aid digestion and reduce kapha and vata. Pitta types should avoid eating cloves too often. Cloves contain red energy, which is especially warming in the winter.

600g (1¼ lb) boneless lamb, cubed

2 medium onions, cut into quarters, plus 2 extra onions, sliced

14 cloves garlic, peeled

1 tablespoon sliced ginger

3 fresh green chillies, cut into 2.5-cm (1-in) pieces

4 tablespoons sunflower oil

1 tablespoon coriander seed

4 cloves

10 black peppercorns

5 fresh red chillies, deseeded

¼ teaspoon fenugreek seed

2-cm (¾-in) piece of fresh ginger, crushed

2 tomatoes, chopped

½ teaspoon ground turmeric

sea salt

1 teaspoon tamarind pulp, diluted in 3 teaspoons water

Preparation time: 20 minutes
Cooking time: 45 minutes plus small bamboo skewers, soaked in water for a couple of hours before using
Serves: 4

1 Thread the lamb, quartered onion, 10 of the garlic cloves, ginger and green chilli on to the skewers alternately to make ribbons of colour. Set aside.

2 Heat 1 tablespoon of the oil in a kadhai or deep frying pan or skillet, and fry the coriander seed, cloves, peppercorns, red chillies and fenugreek seed until they turn golden.

3 Add the sliced onion and fry until brown. Crush the remaining 4 garlic cloves and combine with the crushed ginger to make a paste. Add to the onion mixture, along with the chopped tomatoes, and cook for about 5 minutes. Remove from the heat, cool slightly and blend or process to a paste.

4 Heat the remaining 3 tablespoons oil until almost smoking in a flat, deep pan. Sprinkle with the turmeric. Place the prepared skewers in the oil, turning them to cook the meat evenly on all sides.

5 Add the ground paste, salt to taste and 300 ml (1¼ cups) hot water. Bring to a boil, then simmer until the lamb is cooked, about 30 minutes.

6 Stir in the tamarind juice and remove from the heat.

7 Serve with rice or Flatbread (see page 100) and a fresh green salad.

Sesame Lamb

This sweet, sour and spicy dish is finished with roasted sesame seeds, which add a nutty flavour and provide texture. Sesame seeds are considered hot and heavy, and in North India during winter they are cooked in sugar and eaten to counteract the biting cold. Toasted sesame seeds are best for vata. Sesame oil is wonderful as a skin lubricant for dry winter skin.

1 tablespoon each freshly crushed ginger and garlic, combined (see page 18)

1½ tablespoons jaggery or dark soft brown sugar

600 g (1¼ lb) lean boneless lamb, cubed

1 tablespoon poppy seed

½ teaspoon cardamom seed

1 teaspoon aniseed

½ teaspoon ground cinnamon

4 tablespoons sunflower oil

1 teaspoon mustard seed

1 teaspoon chilli powder

1 teaspoon ground turmeric

1 teaspoon ground coriander

sea salt

1 teaspoon toasted sesame seed

Preparation time: **15 minutes** plus **1 hour** for marinating
Cooking time: **55 minutes**
Serves: **4**

1 Combine the ginger-garlic paste and jaggery, and smear the mixture over the lamb. Marinate in the refrigerator for an hour.

2 Heat a shallow frying pan or skillet, and dry-roast the poppy seed, cardamom seed and aniseed for a couple of minutes. Add the cinnamon and remove from the heat.

3 Blend or process to a fine powder and set aside.

4 Heat the oil until almost smoking in a heavy-bottomed pan and add the mustard seed. When the seeds start to crackle, add the chilli powder, turmeric, coriander and marinated lamb. Add salt to taste, and stir-fry for 10 minutes, taking care not to scorch the sugar.

5 Sprinkle in the poppy seed powder and pour in 300 ml (1¼ cups) hot water. Bring to a boil. Reduce the heat and cook, adding a little more water as necessary, until the lamb is cooked and fairly dry, about 40 minutes.

6 Serve hot, sprinkled with sesame seeds. This dish goes well with Flatbread (see page 100) or Mung Bean Pancakes (see page 105).

Lamb with Ripe Mango

Ripe mangoes are balancing to each of the doshas and contain high amounts of vitamins A and C, which tone the tissues and build immunity. They are heating and can upset the digestion if eaten in excess. I always choose soft, pulpy mangoes for this recipe and take care not to use any variety that is too fibrous. This is a wonderful dish when you are chilled or tired, as the mango provides warmth evenly over a period of a few hours, making you feel content and relaxed.

4 tablespoons sunflower oil

4 cardamoms, crushed

2.5-cm (1-in) piece of cinnamon stick

3 fresh green chillies, slit lengthways

½ tablespoon each freshly crushed ginger and garlic, combined (see page 18)

600 g (1¼ lb) lean boneless lamb, cut into strips

1 teaspoon ground turmeric

sea salt

150 g (5 oz) ripe mango, peeled and grated

150 ml (²/₃ cup) natural (plain) yoghurt, diluted in 150 ml (²/₃ cup) water

1 tablespoon freshly chopped coriander (cilantro) leaves

Preparation time: 15 minutes
Cooking time: 50 minutes
Serves: 4

1 Heat the oil until almost smoking in a heavy-bottomed pan, and fry the cardamom and cinnamon for a minute. Add the chilli and ginger-garlic paste, and stir a couple of times.

2 Next add the lamb and fry for about 10 minutes until browned. Sprinkle with the turmeric and salt to taste. Stir through.

3 Tip in the mango and mix well. Pour in the diluted yoghurt – diluting the yoghurt makes it more compatible with mango.

4 Bring to a boil, reduce the heat, cover and cook until done, about 30 minutes. Add a little water if necessary to prevent the curry from drying out. Sprinkle with the coriander.

5 Serve hot, with Flatbread (see page 100) and Fresh Dill Potatoes (see page 81) for some rejuvenating green energy.

Fragrant Lamb with Green Beans

The red energy of meat is tempered by the green energy of the beans, raising the nutritive value of this dish. The fresher the beans, the more effective they will be; all of the doshas respond well to them. However, undercooking green beans can increase vata. They are also used as a diuretic. Retain their wonderful colour by cooking them without covering the pan.

2 tablespoons sunflower oil

1 teaspoon cumin seed

600 g (1¼ lb) lamb mince (ground lamb)

1 teaspoon ground turmeric

1 teaspoon chilli powder

1 teaspoon garam masala

150 g (5 oz) fresh green beans, halved

2 fresh tomatoes, diced

sea salt

Preparation time: **15 minutes**
Cooking time: **35 minutes**
Serves: **4**

1 Heat the oil until almost smoking in a heavy-bottomed pan and drop in the cumin seed. When the seeds darken slightly, add the lamb and stir-fry for 10 minutes.

2 Add the turmeric, chilli powder, garam masala and beans, stir through and cook for 10 minutes.

3 Next add the tomato and salt to taste, and cook until the lamb and beans are done, about 10-15 minutes.

4 Serve hot, with Cornbread (see page 104) and Lentils with Onion & Cumin (see page 87).

PHALI
KEEMA

Lamb & Potato Patties

Potatoes provide easy-to-digest starch in a meat dish and, thanks to their lightness, they are good for kapha and pitta. They can, however, aggravate vata unless combined with a little heavy fat such as butter or oil. I heve used purple-skinned potatoes (such as Desiree or purple Congo) in this recipe, as they contain a balance of both blue and red energy. Consequently, they are beautifully nourishing without being excessively stimulating. Violet vibrations also help to relax the central nervous system.

3 tablespoons sunflower oil, plus extra for shallow-frying

1 teaspoon ground turmeric

1 teaspoon chilli powder

1 teaspoon garam masala

300 g (10 oz) lean lamb mince (ground lamb)

½ tablespoon each freshly crushed ginger and garlic, combined (see page 18)

1 medium onion, finely chopped

300 g (10 oz) red- or purple-skinned potatoes, boiled, peeled and mashed

4 tablespoons freshly chopped coriander (cilantro) leaves

2 tablespoons freshly chopped mint leaves

sea salt

Preparation time: 20 minutes
Cooking time: 45 minutes
Serves: 4

1 Heat the oil until almost smoking in a heavy-bottomed pan, and tip in the turmeric, chilli powder and garam masala. Immediately add the mince and ginger-garlic paste.

2 Stir-fry for 10–15 minutes, adjusting the heat to avoid burning, until the lamb is cooked. Remove from the heat and mix in the remaining ingredients except the extra sunflower oil, to make a stiff dough. Chill for 15 minutes.

3 Make 8 equal-sized balls of the mixture. Flatten and set aside.

4 Heat the extra oil in a shallow frying pan or skillet, and gently place the patties in it. Fry until the bottoms are crisp and golden, then turn and cook on the other side.

5 Serve hot, with tomato ketchup and a fresh green salad.

Minted Roast Lamb

The green energy of mint helps to strengthen the heart and lower lungs. It is cooling in nature and tempers the heat of lamb, making this dish more acceptable for all of the doshas. It is especially good for bringing pitta into balance and will be even more effective as a lunchtime dish because pitta is most fiery at high noon. This dish will help to calm irritability, anger and frustration, all traits that are typical of this dosha.

½ leg of lamb, fillet end, about 600 g (1 ¼ lb)

sea salt

2 medium onions, quartered

2 fresh green chillies

large handful of fresh mint leaves

3 cloves garlic

2 tablespoons freshly squeezed lemon juice

3 tablespoons honey

2 tablespoons ghee (see page 124)

Preparation time: **15 minutes**
Cooking time: **Approximately 1 ½ hours,**
depending on size of lamb leg
Serves: **4**

1 Preheat the oven to 190°C (375°F, gas mark 5). Make 6-8 incisions in the leg of lamb and rub with salt. Set aside.

2 Blend or process the onions, chillies, mint and garlic to a paste. Combine with the lemon juice and honey.

3 Smear the meat with the mint puree. Place in a roasting tin (pan) with the ghee and cook for 30 minutes to the pound.

4 When the lamb is cooked, transfer it to a serving dish, drain off the fat and collect the juices to serve with the 'raan', or roast.

5 Serve with a bright mango and orange chutney and hot Flatbread (see page 100).

PUDINA

RAAN

Lamb Mince with Aubergine

There are two schools of thought in ayurveda about the potency of aubergine (eggplant). Indian aubergines (these are usually small, greenish purple and have many seeds) are considered heating, whereas those found outside India (normally large, dark-skinned and fleshier) are cooling. Both are light and therefore useful for kapha. Vata can handle them if well spiced, and pitta tolerates them if they are eaten in moderation. Aubergines should not be eaten when you are recovering from an operation or any physical injury, as they are felt to hamper healing.

1 large plump aubergine (eggplant), about 300 g (10 oz)

3 tablespoons sunflower oil

1 medium onion, finely chopped

2 fresh green chillies, chopped

½ tablespoon each freshly crushed ginger and garlic, combined (see page 18)

1 teaspoon ground coriander

1 tablespoon garam masala

1 tablespoon tomato puree (paste)

350 g (12 oz) lean lamb mince (ground lamb)

sea salt

1 tablespoon freshly chopped coriander (cilantro) leaves

Preparation time: 10 minutes
Cooking time: 40 minutes
Serves: 4

1 Hold the aubergine directly over a gas flame and roast until the flesh is pulpy and the skin blackened and crisp. If you do not have a gas burner, use a grill or broiler, keeping the aubergine close to the heat source. You will need to turn it, holding the stalk, from time to time. Cool under cold, running water, peel off and discard the skin and mash the flesh with a fork. Set aside.

2 Heat the oil until almost smoking in a heavy-bottomed pan, and fry the onion until golden. Add the chilli and ginger-garlic paste. Stir through.

3 Sprinkle in the ground coriander and garam masala, and add the tomato puree. Stir over a low heat for 5 minutes.

4 Add the lamb and salt to taste, and stir-fry until cooked, about 15 minutes. Add the reserved aubergine and mix well. Sprinkle the chopped coriander over the top.

5 Serve hot with Millet Bread (see page 103) and Pomegranate Seeds Tossed in Spices (see page 113).

KEEMA BAINGAN

Almond & Raisin Lamb Curry

Nuts, especially almonds, are considered warm and restorative according to ayurvedic principles, and they are used extensively as a tonic for the nerves. They are used blanched as their skins are difficult to digest. Raisins, too, are one of ayurveda's oldest remedies and are used to cure any number of conditions from constipation to toxic imbalances. When soaked in a little water, they are balancing to all of the doshas. Their indigo colour is linked with the nervous system and, consequently, raisins help us to overcome fears and inhibitions.

4 tablespoons sunflower oil

600 g (1¼ lb) lean boneless lamb, cut into strips

2 tablespoons raisins, soaked in water

4 tablespoons blanched almonds, coarsely pounded

1 tablespoon garam masala

1 teaspoon chilli powder

sea salt

300 ml (1¼ cups) natural (plain) yoghurt, beaten

Preparation time: **15 minutes**
Cooking time: **45 minutes**
Serves: **4**

1 Heat the oil in a heavy-bottomed pan and add the lamb. Brown well.

2 Drain the raisins, discarding the soaking water, and add to the meat with the almonds.

3 Add the garam masala, chilli powder and salt to taste. Stir well, then pour in 150 ml (⅔ cup) hot water. Bring to a boil and simmer for about 10 minutes.

4 Next add the yoghurt and cook for a further 10 minutes, until the lamb is cooked. Serve hot, with Flatbread (see page 100) and Cucumber & Dill Salad (see page 108).

SALAN-E-NAAZ

Vegetables

Most of us no longer give credence to the myth that a vegetarian diet lacks adequate proteins or essential minerals and vitamins. In fact, vegetarian protein is far more easily digestible than meat protein, thus taxing the body less and allowing energy to be used for activities other than the process of digestion. And while a big meal of meat can make you feel lethargic, a large meal of vegetables can seem light and yet be filled with energy.

Ayurvedic cooking aims to preserve the vital life force, or prana, of food. Fresh, organic foods are full of this powerful force.

Potatoes with Green Peas

Ayurveda recommends a largely vegetarian diet, which is considered to be sattvic, or one that purifies the body and quietens the mind. Sattvic food, when cooked in the prescribed manner and not greatly spiced or oily, is ideal for everybody, whatever their dosha. Green peas are cool and heavy in nature and do wonders for both pitta and kapha. They need to be spiced for vata, as they have a tendency to cause wind.

1 tablespoon sunflower oil

1 teaspoon cumin seed

½ teaspoon freshly grated ginger

pinch of asafoetida powder

5 curry leaves

2 fresh green chillies, slit lengthways

½ teaspoon ground turmeric

150 g (5 oz) fresh or frozen green peas

2 large tomatoes, grated

sea salt

2 large waxy potatoes, about 300 g (10 oz), boiled, peeled and diced

small handful of fresh coriander (cilantro) leaves, to garnish (optional)

Preparation time: **10 minutes**
Cooking time: **25 minutes**
Serves: 4

1 Heat the oil until almost smoking in a heavy-bottomed pan, and fry the cumin seeds until they turn brown.

2 Add the ginger, asafoetida, curry leaves, chilli and turmeric, and stir through.

3 Next add the peas, tomato and salt to taste, and cook for 5 minutes.

4 Pour in 300ml (1¼ cups) hot water, bring to a boil and reduce the heat. Simmer for 15 minutes, uncovered, until the vegetables are cooked. Add the potato and adjust the seasoning.

5 Serve hot, sprinkled with a dash of coriander, if wished.

ALOO
MATTAR

Cauliflower with Coconut

The cabbage family, to which cauliflower belongs, is best suited to pitta and kapha. It really should be avoided by vata because some members of this family, cauliflower among them, are cold and heavy, and need a good, roaring agni to digest them. Vata tolerates cauliflower better when it is cooked and spiced, as in this recipe. For those blessed with a strong digestion, this vegetable is a good source of bulk and fibre. Its green energy provides a sense of balance.

3 tablespoons sunflower oil

4 black peppercorns

2 cloves

1 tablespoon coriander seed

1 small onion, chopped

150 g (5 oz) fresh coconut, grated, or desiccated (shredded) coconut

500 g (1 lb) cauliflower, cut into florets

1 teaspoon ground turmeric

½ teaspoon chilli powder

2 large tomatoes, chopped

sea salt

Preparation time: **15 minutes**
Cooking time: **25 minutes**
Serves: 4

1 Heat 1 tablespoon of the oil until almost smoking in a heavy-bottomed pan, and fry the peppercorns, cloves and coriander seed for a minute.

2 Add the onion and stir until brown. Stir in the coconut and continue to brown.

3 Remove from the heat, cool slightly and blend or process to a paste with a little water. Set aside.

4 Heat the remaining 2 tablespoons oil until almost smoking in a deep-sided pan, and stir-fry the cauliflower for a couple of minutes. Add the turmeric, chilli powder, tomato and salt to taste, and gently stir-fry for a further 5 minutes.

5 Pour in 150 ml (⅔ cup) hot water and bring to a boil. Add the reserved coconut paste and simmer until the cauliflower is cooked but still firm, about 10–12 minutes.

6 Serve hot, with Millet Bread (see page 103) and Lentils with Onion & Cumin (see page 87).

Spinach with Cottage Cheese

Indian cottage cheese is known as paneer. It is marvellously cooling for pitta, while vata finds its moist heaviness balancing. It is too heavy for kapha to eat regularly, but it is definitely a healthier option than many hard cheeses which are even heavier to digest and therefore more aggravating to this dosha. In colour therapy, paneer is considered to have green energy as it is made of milk, which is generated from grass. It can be nourishing for people fighting cysts or tumours, or any similar cellular malfunction.

500 g (1 lb) fresh spinach, washed and drained

3 tablespoons sunflower oil

½ teaspoon cumin seed

2 large onions, grated

½ tablespoon each freshly crushed ginger and garlic, combined (see page 18)

2 tomatoes, chopped

½ teaspoon chilli powder

½ teaspoon garam masala

sea salt

250 g (8 oz) paneer or firm cottage cheese*, cut into cubes

2 tablespoons single (light) or double (heavy) cream

Preparation time: **10 minutes**
Cooking time: **25 minutes**
Serves: **4**

1 Put the spinach and some water in a heavy saucepan, and cook, uncovered, over a high heat until done, about 10 minutes. Cool slightly, then blend or process until roughly chopped. Set aside.

2 Heat the oil until almost smoking in a heavy-bottomed pan, and fry the cumin seed until brown. Add the onion and fry until the onion is translucent and all the juice has evaporated.

3 Stir in the ginger–garlic paste and tomato, and cook over a low heat until mushy, about 5 minutes.

4 Pour in the spinach puree, sprinkle in the chilli powder, garam masala and salt to taste, and stir well. Bring to a boil.

5 Reduce the heat and add the cubed paneer. Simmer for a minute, then remove from the heat.

6 Serve hot, with the cream swirled on top. This is great with Flatbread (see page 100) and Carrot & Raisin Salad (see page 110).

* If you cannot find paneer or a cottage cheese suitable for dicing, substitute with a mild-flavoured soft white cheese that is firm enough to hold its shape at least a little.

PALAK PANEER

Doodhi with Lentils

Doodhi is a long, pale green vegetable belonging to the gourd family. It is moist and easy to digest, and it makes a wonderful meal for pitta on a hot summer day. Vata and kapha, too, are balanced when this vegetable is served warmly spiced as in this recipe. The green energy of doodhi is anti-ageing and keeps you energetic and focused. If you cannot buy doodhi, marrow or summer squash makes a good substitute.

3 tablespoons channa dal (split dried chickpeas)

2 tablespoons sunflower oil

1 teaspoon cumin seed

pinch of asafoetida powder

½ teaspoon ground turmeric

1 medium doodhi or marrow, about 300 g (10 oz), peeled and diced

1 teaspoon ground coriander

1 teaspoon freshly grated ginger

sea salt

1 tablespoon freshly chopped coriander (cilantro) leaves

Preparation time: 15 minutes plus overnight soaking
Cooking time: 30 minutes
Serves: 4

1 Rinse the channa dal in several changes of cold water, then soak overnight in fresh cold water.

2 Drain the soaked dal, rinse and put in a heavy saucepan. Cover with 300 ml (1¼ cups) hot water. Bring to a boil, reduce the heat and simmer until soft, about 15 minutes – the length of time will depend on the quality of the dal. Set aside.

3 In the meantime, heat the oil until almost smoking in a heavy-bottomed pan, and fry the cumin seed until brown. Add the asafoetida, turmeric and doodhi, and stir through.

4 Add the ground coriander, ginger and salt to taste, and mix well. Pour in 150 ml (⅔ cup) hot water, and bring to a boil. Reduce the heat, cover and simmer for 10 minutes. Add the reserved chana dal and chopped coriander.

5 Serve hot, with Potato-stuffed Bread (see page 101) and a fresh green salad.

Fenugreek Leaves with Potato & Tomato

Fenugreek leaves are slightly bitter in taste, but are rich in vitamin A, which fortifies the mucous membranes, and calcium for good teeth and iron. They help to stimulate agni, but can cause slight constipation. This is why they are usually combined with potatoes, which are an easily digested starchy food and have the extra advantage of adding bulk. Fenugreek balances kapha, but aggravates pitta unless it is cooked properly; it can be tolerated by vata in moderation.

bunch of fenugreek leaves, about 300 g (10 oz)

1 tablespoon sunflower oil

½ teaspoon cumin seed

2 large potatoes, about 250 g (8 oz), washed and diced

¼ teaspoon chilli powder

1 teaspoon ground coriander

2 large tomatoes, chopped

sea salt

Preparation time: **15 minutes**
Cooking time: **25 minutes**
Serves: **4**

1 Pinch the leaves off the fenugreek, discarding the thick central stalks. Rinse, drain and chop the leaves. Set aside.

2 Heat the oil until almost smoking in a heavy-bottomed pan, and fry the cumin seed until brown. Add the remaining ingredients, including the reserved fenugreek. Mix well.

3 Pour in 300 ml (1¼ cups) hot water, and bring to a boil. Reduce the heat, and simmer for about 20 minutes until the potato is tender.

4 Serve hot, with Mung Bean Pancakes (see page 105).

Broccoli in Creamy Coconut Milk

Broccoli is the lightest member of the cabbage family. It is easy to digest, although people with a vata constitution, who are often beleaguered by gas, can tolerate it only very occasionally. It is wonderfully balancing for pitta and kapha, and brings a rich treasure of vitamins to the table, especially A and C. The green of broccoli provides comfort and helps to diminish stress levels.

2 tablespoons sunflower oil

½ teaspoon mustard seed

½ teaspoon cumin seed

pinch of asafoetida powder

1 fresh green chilli, slit lengthways

5 curry leaves

1 medium onion, grated

300 g (10 oz) broccoli florets

300 ml (1 ¼ cups) coconut milk

sea salt

Preparation time: 15 minutes
Cooking time: 20 minutes
Serves: 4

1 Heat the oil until almost smoking, and fry the mustard seed until the seeds begin to pop. Add the cumin seed and fry until brown.

2 Add the asafoetida, chilli, curry leaves and onion. Fry for 5 minutes over a low heat.

3 Tip in the broccoli and cook, uncovered, for 10 minutes, stirring occasionally.

4 Pour in the coconut milk, season with salt to taste and bring to just under a boil. Reduce the heat and simmer for 5-7 minutes until the vegetable is tender but still retains a bite.

5 Serve hot with Potato-stuffed Bread (see page 101) and Sesame Lamb (see page 53) .

BROCCOLI

MALAI

Mushrooms in a Tangy Yoghurt Curry

Mushrooms are inherently dry and cool, and agree with pitta and kapha. They become suitable for vata when they are spiced or, as in this recipe, cooked in a heavy, moist sauce. Kapha types can use soya yoghurt to make this recipe acceptable, while pitta should dilute the yoghurt with water. This dish combines the blue energy of mushrooms with the green energy of yoghurt to promote restfulness and good sleep.

2 tablespoons sunflower oil

2 cloves

2 green cardamom pods, crushed

2.5-cm (1-in) piece of cinnamon stick

½ teaspoon cumin seed

½ teaspoon fennel seed

300 g (10 oz) mushrooms, cleaned and quartered

300 ml (1¼ cups) natural (plain) yoghurt, beaten

sea salt

Preparation time: **15 minutes**
Cooking time: **15 minutes**
Serves: **4**

1 Heat the oil until almost smoking in a heavy saucepan, and fry the cloves, cardamom, cinnamon, cumin seed and fennel seed for a minute or so.

2 Add the mushrooms and stir-fry for a couple of minutes more.

3 Pour in the yoghurt, add salt to taste and cook for a further 10 minutes, lowering the heat when the curry starts to bubble.

4 Serve hot, accompanied by Boiled Rice (see page 96).

KHUMB YAKHNI

Okra in a Velvet Buttermilk Sauce

Okra grows best in a tropical climate, so you will probably find only imported okra in most Western countries. In this case, it is doubly essential that you buy the vegetable as fresh as possible. A sure test is to snap the pointed end; if it breaks crisply the okra is fresh. Any elasticity indicates poor quality. Here the okra is cooked in buttermilk, which tones the digestive tract. This dish is agreeable in small quantities to pitta and kapha (use soya yoghurt for the latter), but make sure that you add the asafoetida powder to warm it up for vata.

2 tablespoons sunflower oil

1 teaspoon mustard seed

½ teaspoon cumin seed

¼ teaspoon fenugreek seed

pinch of asafoetida powder

½ teaspoon ground turmeric

½ teaspoon chilli powder

300 g (10 oz) fresh okra, tops cut off, sliced lengthways

sea salt

300 ml (1¼ cups) natural (plain) yoghurt, beaten

4 tablespoons besan (chickpea flour)

Preparation time: **20 minutes**
Cooking time: **25 minutes**
Serves: **4**

1 Heat the oil until almost smoking in a heavy-bottomed pan, and fry the mustard seed until the seeds begin to pop.

2 Add the cumin seed, fenugreek seed and asafoetida. Sprinkle in the turmeric and chilli powder.

3 Next add the okra and season with salt to taste. Leave over a low heat, stirring occasionally.

4 In the meantime, beat together the yoghurt and flour, along with 300 ml (1¼ cups) cold water, until there are no lumps. Pour the yoghurt mixture over the okra and bring to a boil. Reduce the heat and simmer for 10 minutes until done.

5 Serve hot, with Boiled Rice (see page 96).

DAHI BHINDI

Garden Vegetables in a Tomato Curry

Turmeric, prized for its rich golden colour, has the ability to bring together and blend all the other flavours in a curry. It has long been valued as a blood purifier and antiseptic. Turmeric helps to digest proteins more completely, so that fewer toxins are produced. In India a home remedy for burns or cuts is to apply a little turmeric to the affected area. It is also used in face masks to treat acne or pimples.

3 large tomatoes, grated and skins discarded

2 tablespoons besan (chickpea flour)

2 tablespoons sunflower oil

1 teaspoon mustard seed

¼ teaspoon fenugreek seed

6 curry leaves

1 teaspoon freshly grated ginger

300 g (10 oz) mixed fresh garden vegetables (such as carrots, green beans, green peas, potatoes), peeled and diced

1 teaspoon ground turmeric

½ teaspoon chilli powder

1 teaspoon ground coriander

sea salt

Preparation time: **15 minutes**
Cooking time: **25 minutes**
Serves: **4**

1 Beat together the tomato and besan, pouring in 300 ml (1¼ cups) cold water to make a thin mixture. Set aside.

2 Heat the oil until almost smoking in a heavy-bottomed pan, and fry the mustard seed until the seeds begin to pop. Add the fenugreek seed and curry leaves, and allow to darken slightly.

3 Add the ginger and vegetables, along with the turmeric, chilli powder, coriander and salt to taste. Stir-fry for 5 minutes.

4 Pour in the tomato mixture and bring to a boil, stirring occasionally to prevent sticking. Reduce the heat and simmer for 12-15 minutes until the vegetables are tender and the sauce has thickened. You may need to add more water to prevent the sauce becoming too thick.

5 Serve hot.

TAMATER KADHI

Green Beans with Corn

Fresh, crisp green beans are well tolerated by all the doshas, and sweetcorn is able to balance both vata and pitta with its moist juiciness. In ayurveda, ghee is recommended as the best fat to eat because it is light and easy to digest (see page 13). However, I use sunflower oil in much of my cooking, as it leaves no lingering aftertaste and contains little or no cholesterol, which is an important consideration for a healthy heart.

1 tablespoon sunflower oil

½ teaspoon mustard seed

½ teaspoon cumin seed

1 fresh green chilli, slit lengthways

150 g (5 oz) fresh green beans, ends trimmed and cut into 1.5-cm (½-in) pieces

150 g (5 oz) fresh sweetcorn

sea salt

Preparation time: **15 minutes**
Cooking time: **20 minutes**
Serves: **4**

1 Heat the oil until almost smoking in a heavy frying pan or skillet, and fry the mustard seed until the seeds begin to pop. Add the cumin and chilli.

2 Tip in the vegetables and season to taste with salt, then pour in 4 tablespoons water and cook, uncovered, for about 15 minutes or until tender. You may need to add a little water as necessary to prevent the vegetables sticking to the pan.

3 Thoroughly drain the vegetables and serve hot to accompany a chicken curry and rice.

FARASBEE
MAKAI

Spring Onions Tossed in Spices

In spite of their pungency and ability to make your eyes water, white onions are actually cooling and are used in ayurveda to treat a variety of conditions ranging from coughs and colds to fevers. Spring onions are ideal in the summer, and tossing them in spices makes them easier to digest. Their fresh green colour strengthens the energy centre of the heart and lower lungs; emotionally, it promotes a sense of contentment and relaxation.

2 tablespoons sunflower oil

½ teaspoon mustard seed

8–10 curry leaves

pinch of asafoetida powder

300 g (10 oz) spring onions (scallions), chopped

½ teaspoon ground coriander

sea salt

Preparation time: **10 minutes**
Cooking time: **15 minutes**
Serves: **4**

1 Heat the oil until almost smoking in a heavy-bottomed pan, and add the mustard seed. When the seeds begin to pop, add the curry leaves and asafoetida.

2 Add the spring onion, coriander and salt to taste. Stir-fry for 5-7 minutes until the raw smell disappears and the onion begins to soften. Reduce the heat and cook for a further 5 minutes.

3 This makes a wonderful meal accompanied by Flatbread (see page 100) and Curried Black-eyed Beans (see page 90).

KANDYACHI
BHAJI

Spiced Pumpkin

Pumpkin is considered sweet, moist and cool, so on the whole it does not stimulate digestion. Its sweetness will, however, provide a sense of fullness and satisfaction at the end of a meal. To make it more digestible, it must be cooked with warming spices. It is best for vata, increases kapha and can be tolerated by pitta occasionally. It is a rich source of potassium, vital for the proper functioning of the heart, and vitamin A, which is essential for clear vision. Its orange energy is useful in removing inhibitions or restraint, and gives strength of purpose.

300 g (10 oz) pumpkin, peeled and diced

1 tablespoon sunflower oil

½ teaspoon mustard seed

½ teaspoon cumin seed

¼ teaspoon fenugreek seed

¼ teaspoon fennel seed

2 fresh red chillies, slit lengthways and deseeded

sea salt

½ teaspoon granulated sugar

Preparation time: **10 minutes**
Cooking time: **15 minutes**
Serves: **4**

1 Steam the pumpkin in a steamer until just tender, about 7 minutes. Set aside.

2 Heat the oil until almost smoking in a small saucepan, and fry the mustard seed until the seeds begin to pop. Add the cumin, fenugreek and fennel seeds with the chilli, and fry for a few seconds.

3 Quickly pour the oil and spices over the reserved pumpkin. Sprinkle with salt to taste and the sugar, and toss gently to mix.

4 Serve warm, as an accompaniment to Golden Mung Dal (see page 85) and rice.

KADDU

CHORCHORI

Warm Potatoes with Cumin

The most nutritious way of cooking potatoes is without peeling them, as most of the vitamins and minerals lie in or just under their skins. Potatoes must be treated with great caution because they belong to the deadly nightshade family and can be the bearers of an alarming store of toxins. This can show up as a greenish tinge on or near the peel, which must be cut off before use, or as a burning taste on the tongue. This is an indication of high alkaloid levels that can be toxic. In this recipe the cumin helps to expel any residual toxins.

**4 large potatoes, about 500 g (1 lb),
boiled in their skins**

sea salt

1 tablespoon sunflower oil

1 teaspoon cumin seed

½ teaspoon ground turmeric

½ teaspoon chilli powder

Preparation time: **5 minutes**
Cooking time: **25 minutes**
Serves: **4**

1 Cut the potatoes into cubes and sprinkle with salt. Set aside.

2 Heat the oil until almost smoking in a heavy-bottomed pan, and fry the cumin seed until it starts to brown.

3 Add the turmeric, chilli powder and reserved potatoes. Mix well. Don't worry if the potatoes crumble a little and become slightly mushy.

4 Serve hot as an accompaniment to lamb and boiled or steamed rice.

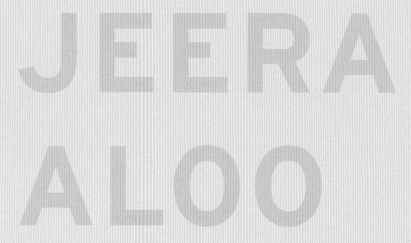

JEERA
ALOO

Mixed Peppers with Cashews

This recipe brings together orange, red and green energy in a great burst, so that it helps to build a good appetite, provide stamina for physical activity and bring balance to all the areas of your life. Cashews are hot and heavy, and can be handled only by vata. Pitta and kapha people could omit them in this recipe. The heat of the peppers helps to stimulate agni.

1 teaspoon sunflower oil

½ teaspoon cumin seed

pinch of asafoetida powder

1 small onion, sliced

300 g (10 oz) mixed peppers, quartered, deseeded and sliced

1 teaspoon ground coriander

sea salt

2 tablespoons raw cashew nuts

1 teaspoon freshly squeezed lemon juice

Preparation time: **15 minutes**
Cooking time: **10 minutes**
Serves: **4**

1 Heat the oil until almost smoking in a heavy saucepan, and add the cumin seed. When it begins to darken, add the asafoetida and onion.

2 Stir until the onion becomes translucent, then add the peppers, coriander, salt to taste and cashews. Stir for 5 minutes until just softened.

3 Remove the pan from the heat, and mix in the lemon juice.

4 Serve warm, accompanied by Garlic-flavoured Lentils (see page 89) and rice.

KAJU SIMLA MIRCH

Beetroot with Fresh Coriander

Beetroot (red beets) is warm, sweet and moist, and is recommended for those with a sluggish digestion. These beets add bulk and fibre, and have been used to relieve haemorrhoids. They are very rich in folic acid, which helps to keep the blood circulation in prime condition. Indian women eat beetroot to overcome anaemia. Its rich red colour will help you to be assertive, but an excess of red energy can lead to impatience and anger.

1 tablespoon sunflower oil

½ teaspoon mustard seed

¼ teaspoon cumin seed

5 curry leaves

4 large cooked beetroot (red beets), about 500 g (1 lb), cubed

3 tablespoons freshly chopped coriander (cilantro) leaves

1 tablespoon desiccated (shredded) coconut

Preparation time: **10 minutes**
Cooking time: **5 minutes**
Serves: **4**

1 Heat the oil until almost smoking in a saucepan, and fry the mustard seed until the seeds begin to pop. Add the cumin seed and curry leaves.

2 Add the beetroot, coriander and coconut, and toss together. Warm through gently.

3 Serve with Sweet & Sour Lentils (see page 92) and Boiled Rice (see page 96).

BEET UPKARI

Cabbage with Crunchy Peanuts

Cabbage is very good for most people with a kapha or pitta constitution, but vata people may find it too cold and heavy. It becomes more acceptable to vata with the addition of spices such as asafoetida and mustard seed. Cabbage contains good amounts of folic acid and vitamin C, and it is believed to help in the prevention of cancer. Peanuts, meanwhile, are nutritious and a gentle laxative, but they can promote gas in vata. They are full of vitamins B and E, iron and zinc, which works on the immune and reproductive systems.

1 tablespoon peanuts

1 tablespoon sunflower oil

½ teaspoon mustard seed

½ teaspoon cumin seed

pinch of asafoetida powder

8 curry leaves

2 fresh green chillies, slit lengthways

300 g (10 oz) cabbage, shredded

sea salt

Preparation time: **15 minutes**
Cooking time: **15 minutes**
Serves: **4**

1 Crush the peanuts roughly using a mortar and pestle, and set aside.

2 Heat the oil until almost smoking in a heavy-bottomed pan, and fry the mustard seed until the seeds begin to pop.

3 Add the cumin, asafoetida powder, curry leaves and chilli. Stir through, then add the cabbage and salt to taste. Cook, uncovered, stirring occasionally until the cabbage is nearly cooked but still has a little bite, about 10-12 minutes.

4 Mix in the reserved peanuts and serve warm, with Flatbread (see page 100) and Coriander Dal (see page 88).

KOBICHI BHAJI

Stuffed Aubergines

Aubergines (eggplant) are sweet and oily, and therefore should be cooked with the least amount of oil possible, but a fair amount of spices. The small, round aubergines used in this recipe are heating in effect and are therefore combined with cooling coconut and coriander (cilantro) leaves. Aubergines carry the violet energy ray and, as a result, are associated with the pituitary gland and with intuition and spiritual awareness.

8 small round aubergines (eggplant)

4 tablespoons shredded fresh coconut or desiccated (shredded) coconut

½ teaspoon ground turmeric

½ teaspoon chilli powder

1 teaspoon ground coriander

sea salt

pinch of granulated sugar

2 tablespoons besan (chickpea flour)

2 tablespoons sunflower oil

1 teaspoon mustard seed

Preparation time: **15 minutes**
Cooking time: **30 minutes**
Serves: **4**

1 Slit each aubergine into quarters from the bottom to halfway down, keeping the stem intact so that the vegetable does not fall apart.

2 Combine the coconut, turmeric, chilli powder, coriander, salt to taste, sugar and besan.

3 Stuff the aubergines with the coconut mixture and set aside.

4 Heat the oil until almost smoking in a heavy-bottomed pan and add the mustard seed. As the seeds begin to pop, place the aubergines in the oil and cook for 5 minutes, turning from time to time.

5 Pour in 60 ml (¼ cup) hot water, cover and cook over a low heat until the aubergines are cooked through, about 20 minutes. You may need to add more water to prevent the aubergines sticking to the pan. The final dish should be tender and moist.

6 Serve hot, with Millet Bread (see page 103) and Tropical Pineapple & Coconut Salad (see page 117).

MASALA RINGNA

Courgettes with Lentils

Courgettes (zucchini) are members of the marrow family and are light, cool and easy to digest. They balance vata and pitta beautifully, but can be aggravating to kapha. They are good for people who need to add bulk and fibre to their diet. Courgettes are full of wonderful green energy and have an alkalizing effect on the body. Their rich colour strengthens our links with the earth, attuning us to the positive vibrations in the environment.

2 tablespoons sunflower oil

½ teaspoon cumin seed

8 curry leaves

pinch of asafoetida powder

1 tablespoon urad dal (split black lentils), rinsed and soaked in water for 10 minutes

300 g (10 oz) courgettes (zucchini), cubed

½ teaspoon ground turmeric

½ teaspoon ground coriander

sea salt

1 tablespoon freshly squeezed lemon juice

Preparation time: **10 minutes**
Cooking time: **15 minutes**
Serves: **4**

1 Heat the oil until almost smoking in a heavy-bottomed pan, and fry the cumin seed until it starts to darken.

2 Add the curry leaves, asafoetida and urad dal, and stir for 2 minutes.

3 Tip in the courgettes, turmeric, coriander and salt to taste, and mix well.

4 Cook, uncovered, stirring from time to time until done but still a bit crunchy, about 10 minutes. You could add a tablespoon of water to hasten cooking.

5 Sprinkle with lemon juice and serve hot, accompanied by rice and Whole Red Lentils with Onion & Yoghurt (see page 86).

COURGETTE
BHAJI

Bananas Stuffed with Coriander Chutney

Ripe bananas are cooling, heavy and sweet, although their long-term effect is sour. This makes them a difficult food for kapha and poor for pitta if eaten in excess. They are, however, good for heartburn, gas and inflammations of the gastrointestinal tract. Ripe bananas are used as a remedy for diarrhoea, even in children, or for putting on weight. Their yellow energy is wonderful for the brain and nervous system.

2 tablespoons shredded fresh coconut or desiccated (shredded) coconut

2 tablespoons fresh coriander (cilantro) leaves

¼ teaspoon each freshly crushed ginger and garlic, combined (see page 18)

1 fresh green chilli

sea salt

2 large ripe bananas

2 tablespoons sunflower oil

½ teaspoon mustard seed

Preparation time: 15 minutes
Cooking time: 10 minutes
Serves: 4

1 Blend or process the coconut, coriander, ginger-garlic paste, chilli and salt to taste to a fine paste.

2 Peel the bananas and slit each one into four sections down the middle, leaving the base intact. Put a little of the coriander chutney down the centre of each banana.

3 Heat the oil until almost smoking in a heavy saucepan, and fry the mustard seed until the seeds begin to pop. Carefully add the bananas and cook, turning from time to time for 7-10 minutes until golden brown.

4 Serve hot, accompanied by Flatbread (see page 100) and a spicy dish such as Cauliflower with Coconut (see page 63).

CHUTNEYCHI KELI

Fresh Dill Potatoes

Potatoes are rich in vitamin C and will help to ward off seasonal chills and colds. Dill is a gentle herb that is balancing to all the doshas. The yellow hue of potatoes is associated with all things bright and beautiful – perhaps that is why so many of us consider the potato to be our ideal comfort food.

3 large potatoes, about 300 g (10 oz), boiled in their skins

2 tablespoons sunflower oil

pinch of asafoetida powder

pinch of ground turmeric

1 teaspoon ground coriander

4 teaspoons freshly chopped dill

sea salt

Preparation time: **10 minutes**
Cooking time: **25 minutes**
Serves: **4**

1 Peel the potatoes and cut into cubes. Set aside.

2 Heat the oil until almost smoking in a heavy saucepan, and add the asafoetida, turmeric and coriander.

3 Add the potato, dill and salt to taste. Stir to warm through, then remove from the heat.

4 Serve hot, with Flatbread (see page 100) and lentils.

HARE

BHARE

ALOO

Sprouts,
Lentils
& Beans

In India, where many people are vegetarian, lentils and pulses provide the protein element of the daily diet. Beans are cooked in curry to accompany rice or are sprouted and treated as 'vegetables' to be stir-fried with herbs and spices. Lentils are rich in mineral salts, especially phosphorus and iron.

On the whole, lentils and beans produce heat in the body and need to be teamed with cooling ingredients to balance them. Many traditional recipes combine them with rice and vegetables to make wholesome, one-pot suppers. Lentils are always served with rice or a variety of Indian flatbread known as roti.

Stir-fried Mung Bean Sprouts

The process of sprouting induces a riot of biochemical changes in which complex components break down into simpler substances that are easy to digest. Sprouted legumes contain higher amounts of vitamin C, iron and calcium than those that are unsprouted. Mung bean sprouts, in particular, are slightly cooling and provide positive energy for pitta and vata. Kapha can handle mung beans sprouts in moderation.

150 g (5 oz) dried mung beans

1 tablespoon sunflower oil

½ teaspoon mustard seed

½ teaspoon cumin seed

8 curry leaves

1 small fresh green chilli, slit lengthways

1 medium onion, finely chopped

¼ teaspoon ground turmeric

sea salt

2 tablespoons desiccated (shredded) coconut

1 tablespoon freshly chopped coriander (cilantro) leaves

1 tablespoon freshly squeezed lemon juice

Preparation time: 10 minutes plus 24 hours for soaking and overnight sprouting
Cooking time: 25 minutes
Serves: 4

1 Rinse the mung beans, then soak them in cold water for at least 5 hours. Drain and tie the beans up in a piece of cheesecloth or muslin, then keep in a warm place overnight to sprout. When ready, refresh the sprouted beans in cold water.

2 Heat the oil until almost smoking in a heavy saucepan, and add the mustard. When the seeds begin to pop, add the cumin seed, curry leaves and chilli. Add the onion and fry until translucent.

3 Tip in the sprouted beans, turmeric and salt to taste. Add a little water and cook until the beans are soft but firm, adding more water if necessary.

4 Sprinkle the coconut, coriander and lemon juice over the top. Serve warm.

MUGACHI

USAL

Golden Mung Dal

Mung dal (split mung beans) is highly regarded in ayurveda as it is lighter and easier to digest than most other legumes and pulses. Mung is available as small, dried, whole green beans or split into flattish yellow lentils, called dal, which may be sold with or without the green skins. Mung beans are used in many restorative recipes, as they are cooling and also provide protein and bulk. They are a source of vitamins A, B and C as well.

150 g (5 oz) mung dal (split mung beans), skins on

sea salt

1 tablespoon sunflower oil

pinch of asafoetida powder

1 medium onion, finely chopped

½ teaspoon each freshly crushed ginger and garlic, combined (see page 18)

½ teaspoon ground turmeric

½ teaspoon chilli powder

1 tomato, chopped

Preparation time: 10 minutes plus 1 hour for soaking
Cooking time: **30 minutes**
Serves: **4**

1 Rinse the dal in several changes of water, then leave to soak in fresh cold water for an hour.

2 Put the drained dal in a heavy saucepan with some salt and 300 ml (1¼ cups) hot water. Bring to a boil, reduce the heat and simmer until done, about 20 minutes.

3 Heat the oil until almost smoking in a small saucepan, and add the asafoetida and onion. Cook until golden.

4 Add the ginger-garlic paste, turmeric, chilli powder and tomato, and stir to blend for about 5 minutes. Pour the entire mixture, with the oil, into the cooked dal. Adjust the seasoning, adding a little water if necessary.

5 Serve hot, with Flatbread (see page 100).

CHILKEWALI
MUNG DAL

Whole Red Lentils with Onion & Yoghurt

Red lentils are hot in potency and stimulate agni. People who suffer from gout should be careful with red lentils, as their heat and uric acid content can aggravate the condition. Red lentils are balancing to vata and kapha, but pitta needs to cool them with coriander (cilantro) leaves. Their powerful red energy provides stamina.

150 g (5 oz) whole red lentils

sea salt

1 teaspoon ground turmeric

½ teaspoon chilli powder

1 teaspoon freshly grated ginger

1 tablespoon sunflower oil

½ teaspoon mustard seed

½ teaspoon cumin seed

1 small onion, sliced

2 tablespoons natural (plain) yoghurt

1 tablespoon freshly chopped coriander (cilantro) leaves

Preparation time: 10 minutes plus 1 hour
 for soaking
Cooking time: 45 minutes
Serves: 4

1 Rinse the lentils in several changes of water, then soak them in fresh cold water for an hour to soften them slightly and reduce cooking time.

2 Put the drained lentils, a little salt, turmeric, chilli powder and ginger in a heavy saucepan with 300 ml (1¼ cups) hot water, and bring to a boil. Reduce the heat and simmer until mushy, about 30 minutes.

3 Heat the oil until almost smoking in a small saucepan, and fry the mustard seed until the seeds begin to pop. Add the cumin seed and onion, and fry until the onion is golden and crisp at the edges.

4 Stir in the yoghurt and pour the mixture into the cooked lentils. Adjust the consistency by adding more hot water if necessary.

5 Serve hot, with a sprinkling of coriander. Enjoy with rice and a vegetable stir-fry.

Lentils with Onion & Cumin

The next three recipes are fairly similar in the preparation, but use three distinct flavourings. In this one cumin adds a slightly bitter taste, which relieves pitta as well as kapha. Cumin also helps to stimulate the vata digestion. Cumin seeds are always started off in a little warm oil, as the frying process activates the aromatic oils in the spice. Cumin has long been known as a remedy for excess bile and flatulent colic, while hot cumin water is used as a remedy for colds.

150 g (5 oz) toor dal (split yellow lentils)

1 tablespoon sunflower oil

1 teaspoon cumin seed

pinch of asafoetida powder

1 large onion, chopped

½ teaspoon ground turmeric

sea salt

1 tablespoon freshly squeezed lemon juice

Preparation time: 10 minutes plus 1 hour
   for soaking
Cooking time: 40 minutes
Serves: 4

1 Rinse the lentils in several changes of water, then soak them in fresh cold water for an hour.

2 Put the drained lentils in a heavy saucepan with 300 ml (1¼ cups) hot water and cook until mushy, about 30 minutes.

3 Heat the oil until almost smoking in a small saucepan, and fry the cumin seed until it begins to sizzle. Add the asafoetida powder and onion, and cook until golden.

4 Mix in the turmeric and salt to taste. Pour the mixture into the cooked lentils, and add the lemon juice. Adjust the seasoning, adding a little hot water to thin the consistency if required. Remove from the heat.

5 Serve hot, with rice and a meat curry.

JEERA DAL

Coriander Dal

This fragrant dal is flavoured with fresh coriander (cilantro) leaves. It is balancing to all the doshas and has been used as a diuretic for centuries in India. The cooling leaves are rich in potassium, but asthma sufferers should use coriander sparingly.

150 g (5 oz) toor dal (split yellow lentils)

1 tablespoon sunflower oil

½ teaspoon ground turmeric

pinch of asafoetida powder

2 large tomatoes, grated and skins discarded

sea salt

150 g (5 oz) freshly chopped coriander (cilantro) leaves

Preparation time: 10 minutes plus 1 hour for soaking
Cooking time: 40 minutes
Serves: 4

1 Rinse the lentils in several changes of cold water, then soak them in fresh cold water for an hour.

2 Put the drained lentils in a heavy saucepan with 300 ml (1¼ cups) hot water, and cook until mushy, about 30 minutes.

3 Heat the oil until almost smoking in a small saucepan, and add the turmeric, asafoetida, tomato and salt to taste. Stir briskly until well blended and mushy.

4 Pour the tomato mixture into the cooked lentils and adjust seasoning and consistency, adding hot water if necessary.

5 Stir in the coriander and serve at once, with steamed rice and Spiced Pumpkin (see page 73).

DHANIYE KI DAL

Garlic-flavoured Lentils

Garlic is known as the 'bulb of life' in India. It is hot in potency and calms vata and kapha, but an excess of garlic aggravates pitta. It is used as a winter remedy for arthritis and flu, and is wonderful for sufferers of asthma and other lung conditions. Garlic is also used successfully to reduce high blood pressure.

150 g (5 oz) toor dal (split yellow lentils)

½ teaspoon cumin seed

1 teaspoon ground turmeric

sea salt

1 tablespoon sunflower oil

3 cloves garlic, halved

Preparation time: 10 minutes plus 1 hour
  for soaking
Cooking time: 40 minutes
Serves: 4

1 Rinse the lentils in several changes of cold water, then soak them in fresh cold water for an hour.

2 Put the drained lentils in a heavy saucepan with the cumin seed, turmeric and 350 ml (1½ cups) hot water, and bring to a boil. Reduce the heat and simmer until cooked, about 30 minutes. Remove from the heat, add salt to taste and set aside.

3 Heat the oil until almost smoking in a small saucepan, and fry the garlic until golden. Pour into the lentils and stir through.

4 Serve with Flatbread (see page 100) and Beetroot with Fresh Coriander (see page 76).

LAHSUN KI DAL

Curried Black-eyed Beans

Beans are a valuable food resource not only for humans, but for the earth as well. As crops, they contain nitrogen-fixing bacteria that can draw in large amounts of nitrogen from the atmosphere, convert it into a usable form and release it into the soil in which they grow. This natural fertilization process is invaluable and a vital part of nature's cycle. Black-eyed beans are excellent for pitta and kapha, but can aggravate vata.

150 g (5 oz) black-eyed beans

2 tablespoons sunflower oil

½ teaspoon cumin seed

1 large onion, finely chopped

½ teaspoon each freshly crushed ginger and garlic, combined (see page 18)

1 fresh green chilli, minced

1 teaspoon ground turmeric

1 teaspoon ground coriander

½ teaspoon garam masala

2 large tomatoes, grated and skins discarded

sea salt

1 tablespoon freshly chopped coriander (cilantro) leaves

Preparation time: 15 minutes plus overnight soaking
Cooking time: 40 minutes
Serves: 4

1 Rinse the black-eyed beans in several changes of cold water, then soak overnight in fresh cold water.

2 Heat the oil until almost smoking in a deep, heavy saucepan, and fry the cumin seed until brown.

3 Add the onion and fry until golden, then add the ginger–garlic paste, chilli, turmeric, ground coriander, garam masala and tomato. Stir to soften, about 5 minutes.

4 Now add the black-eyed beans and salt to taste. Pour in 300 ml (1 ¼ cups) hot water and bring to a boil. Reduce the heat and simmer, adding water as necessary to give a pouring consistency, until the beans are tender, about 30 minutes.

5 Serve sprinkled with coriander to accompany Flatbread (see page 100) and a green salad.

LOBHIA KI KADHI

Split Red Lentils with Coconut

Split red lentils are hot in potency, so in this recipe they are combined with coconut to add a cooling touch. Their vibrant red colour affects the kidney and bladder, stimulating and strengthening these organs. Combine this dish with a food from the green spectrum, such as okra or courgettes (zucchini), for a colour-balanced meal.

150 g (5 oz) split red lentils

1 teaspoon sunflower oil

½ teaspoon mustard seed

1 teaspoon cumin seed

pinch of asafoetida powder

½ teaspoon freshly grated ginger

8 curry leaves

2 fresh green chillies, slit lengthways

½ teaspoon ground turmeric

1 large tomato, chopped

sea salt

3 tablespoons shredded coconut

1 tablespoon freshly chopped coriander (cilantro) leaves

Preparation time: 10 minutes plus 1 hour for soaking
Cooking time: 25 minutes
Serves: 4

1 Rinse the lentils in several changes of water, then soak them in fresh cold water for an hour.

2 Set the drained lentils to cook in a heavy saucepan with 300 ml (1¼ cups) hot water. Reduce the heat and simmer for 15 minutes until done.

3 Heat the oil until almost smoking in a small saucepan, and fry the mustard seed until the seeds begin to pop. Add the cumin seed, asafoetida, ginger, curry leaves and chilli. Stir through.

4 Add the turmeric and pour the mixture into the cooked lentils. Next add the tomato, salt to taste and enough water to give a pouring consistency. Simmer for a minute or so.

5 Serve hot, sprinkled with coconut and coriander, accompanied by rice and Spring Onions Tossed in Spices (see page 72).

MASURICHI AMTI

Sweet & Sour Lentils

Tamarind is a dark brown, brittle pod that contains a sticky, sweet-sour pulp. In the West this pulp is sold in jars as a jamlike concentrate. It is hot and heavy, and aggravates kapha and pitta, but is great for vata. It is known to stimulate the digestion and works as a mild laxative. People with blood sugar imbalances should omit the raw cane sugar and add a sautéed onion instead.

150 g (5 oz) split red lentils

1 tablespoon tamarind pulp, diluted in 4 tablespoons water

1 tablespoon raw cane sugar

2 tablespoons roasted peanuts

1 teaspoon ground turmeric

sea salt

2 tablespoons sunflower oil

1 teaspoon mustard seed

large pinch of asafoetida powder

¼ teaspoon fenugreek seed

10 curry leaves

2 tablespoons freshly chopped coriander (cilantro) leaves

Preparation time: **15 minutes plus 1 hour for soaking**
Cooking time: **20 minutes**
Serves: **4**

1 Rinse the lentils in several changes of water, then soak them in fresh cold water for an hour.

2 Put the drained lentils in a heavy saucepan with 300 ml (1¼ cups) hot water, and bring to a boil. Simmer for 15 minutes, then add the tamarind pulp, cane sugar, peanuts, turmeric and salt to taste. Cook for a few more minutes, or until the lentils are done.

3 Heat the oil until almost smoking in a small saucepan, and fry the mustard seed until the seeds begin to pop. Add the asafoetida, fenugreek seed and curry leaves, and pour the mixture into the cooked lentils. Mix well.

4 Serve hot, garnished with coriander. This dal goes well with rice and a vegetable stir-fry.

Black Lentils with Red Beans

The combination of red beans and black lentils is rich and heavy to digest, so is best for those with good agni. Spiced up with asafoetida it is more balancing for vata. Red kidney beans, which benefit pitta, also become more digestible with the addition of spices. Kapha can enjoy this dish occasionally. Black lentils carry the indigo ray, which controls the organs of sight and hearing.

3 tablespoons sunflower oil

1 large onion, grated

½ tablespoon each freshly crushed ginger and garlic, combined (see page 18)

large pinch of asafoetida powder

1 teaspoon ground turmeric

1 teaspoon chilli powder

1 teaspoon garam masala

2 large tomatoes, chopped

150 g (5 oz) whole black lentils

2 tablespoons dried red kidney beans, rinsed well and soaked overnight

sea salt

4 tablespoons double (heavy) cream (omit for pitta and kapha)

2 tablespoons freshly chopped coriander (cilantro) leaves

Preparation time: 15 minutes plus
   overnight soaking
Cooking time: 1 hour 15 minutes
Serves: 4

1 Rinse the lentils in several changes of cold water, then soak them overnight in fresh cold water.

2 Heat the oil until almost smoking in a large, heavy saucepan, and fry the onion until golden. Add the ginger-garlic paste and asafoetida.

3 Stir in the turmeric, chilli powder, garam masala and tomato, and cook for a few minutes to blend.

4 Drain the lentils and beans, and add to the pan with salt to taste. Pour in 300 ml (1¼ cups) hot water and bring to a boil. Reduce the heat and simmer for an hour or until the beans and lentils are cooked. (Dried kidney beans are said to contain a toxic resin that is not destroyed by light cooking, so it is very important that the beans are thoroughly cooked.)

5 Remove from the heat, stir in the cream, if using, and serve garnished with the coriander, accompanied by Boiled Rice (see page 96).

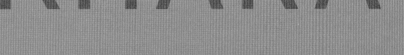

DAL BUKHARA

Rice & Breads

6

Rice is an excellent carbohydrate and one that is very easy to digest. However, the various processes that rice is subjected to in order to make it white and 'beautiful' succeed in removing the outer layer of the grain that contains valuable nutrients such as proteins, lipids, vitamin B and mineral salts. Unpolished rice is considered far more nutritious.

Most Indian breads are made from wholemeal (whole-wheat) flour, which is a healthier alternative than processed white flour. North India grows the majority of the country's wheat. Many towns and villages throughout India have a communal tandoor, or clay oven, in which fresh bread is baked every day.

Boiled Rice

White basmati rice is tridoshic in effect, i.e. it is beneficial to all the doshas. It is fairly cooling, sweet, light and moist. Processing treatments such as polishing through which it passes in order to become visually more appealing deplete it of vital nutrients, but make it more easy to digest and less likely to produce gas than other grains. In ayurveda rice is considered to have yellow energy that suffuses you with a sense of joy.

300 g (2 cups) basmati rice, rinsed and drained

600 ml (2 ½ cups) hot water

sea salt

2 cloves (optional)

Preparation time: **5 minutes**
Cooking time: **up to 30 minutes depending on quality of rice**
Serves: **4**

1 Put all the ingredients in a heavy saucepan and bring to a boil. (I have added the cloves for a touch of warmth, but you can omit these in the summer months.)

2 Reduce the heat, cover partially and simmer until the rice is fluffy and cooked. This may take anything between 15 and 30 minutes, depending on the age and quality of the rice.

3 Gently run a fork through the rice to loosen it, and serve hot with a meat or vegetable curry.

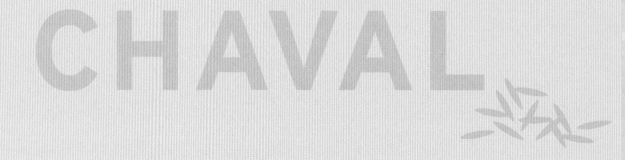

CHAVAL

Rice & Lentil Khichadi

Khichadis are simple combinations of rice, split mung dal and spices, all cooked together until moist and creamy. They are at the heart of panchakarma, or ayurvedic cleansing therapy, as they are easy to digest and assimilate, and also promote lubrication. Various spices are added for specific functions. This recipe is for a digestive khichadi and is often used when a light diet is needed. Its yellow energy adds to the cleansing and digestive effect of the dish.

1 tablespoon ghee (see page 124)

5 cloves

10 black peppercorns

1 bay leaf

½ teaspoon cumin seed

½ teaspoon ground turmeric

300 g (2 cups) basmati rice, rinsed and drained

4 tablespoons mung dal (split mung beans), rinsed and drained

sea salt

Preparation time: **10 minutes**
Cooking time: **35 minutes**
Serves: **4**

1 Heat the ghee until almost smoking in a large, heavy saucepan, and fry the cloves, peppercorns, bay leaf, cumin seed and turmeric for a minute.

2 Add the rice, mung dal, 600 ml (2 ½ cups) hot water and salt to taste, and bring to a boil.

3 Reduce the heat and simmer until the rice is creamy and cooked, about 30 minutes. This dish will be quite moist, which increases its digestibility.

4 Serve with natural (plain) yoghurt.

KHICHADI

Yoghurt Rice

Yoghurt is an excellent digestive and encourages a healthy bacterial balance in the stomach and colon. Vata should finish a meal with a bowl of natural (plain) yoghurt, whereas pitta needs to dilute it with a little water and kapha needs to warm it with spices or mix it with honey. Cucumber is moist, cold and sweet, and is great for vata and pitta, but not for kapha. This dish is suffused with healing green energy.

300 g (2 cups) basmati rice, cooked

300 ml (1 ¼ cups) thick natural (plain) yoghurt

2 tablespoons sunflower oil

1 teaspoon mustard seed

2 dried chillies, deseeded and broken up

10 curry leaves

3 tablespoons chopped cucumber

sea salt

pinch of granulated sugar

Preparation time: **10 minutes**
Cooking time: **25 minutes**
Serves: **4**

1 Mix the cooked rice and yoghurt in a large mixing bowl. Set aside.

2 Heat the oil until almost smoking in a small saucepan, and fry the mustard seed until the seeds begin to pop. Add the chilli and curry leaves, and pour the mixture (including the oil) into the reserved rice.

3 Stir in the cucumber, salt to taste and sugar, and refrigerate before serving.

4 Serve slightly chilled. Hot mango pickle is a perfect partner for this dish.

BAGALA BHATH

Dried Fruit Pulao

This is a festive golden yellow dish dotted with nuts and dried fruit, which provide crunch and flavour. Nuts are full of B vitamins, which help the heart, and folic acid, which promotes healthy hair growth. Dried fruit provides invaluable fibre and energy and importantly contains calcium, which is essential for strong teeth and bones, and it is also a source of iron. Vitamin C is required for the proper absorption of iron, so a squeeze of fresh lemon juice is in order.

1 teaspoon granulated sugar

2 tablespoons sunflower oil

6 green cardamom pods, bruised

6 cloves

2 bay leaves

4 cm (1½ in) cinnamon stick

10 black peppercorns

300 g (2 cups) basmati rice

2 tablespoons raisins

4 tablespoons flaked almonds

4 tablespoons pistachio nuts, chopped

4 tablespoons unsalted cashew nuts

1 teaspoon saffron threads

sea salt

4 tablespoons freshly chopped coriander (cilantro) leaves

4 dried apricots, chopped (to garnish)

squeeze of fresh lemon juice

Preparation time: **15 minutes**
Cooking time: **40 minutes**
Serves: **4**

1 Put the sugar in a heavy-bottomed pan over a high heat and allow it to caramelize. Pour in the oil and blend. When the oil is hot, add the cardamom, cloves, bay leaves, cinnamon and peppercorns, and fry for a minute.

2 Rinse and drain the basmati rice, add to the pan and stir well. Mix in the raisins and half the nuts. Pour in 600 ml (2 ½ cups) hot water, and sprinkle in the saffron and a little salt. Stir and cook over a low heat until the rice is fluffy and dry.

3 Remove from the heat and run a fork through the rice to loosen it.

4 Serve hot, sprinkled with the remaining nuts, coriander and dried apricots. Drizzle with lemon juice. Enjoy with a meat curry and a generous, colourful salad.

Flatbread

Wheat is a cool, heavy, moist grain that contains a substance called aleuron, a mixture of proteins, vitamins and minerals. Modern milling processes destroy this vital substance, so wholemeal (whole-wheat) flour is healthier than the refined variety. Wheat is balancing for vata and pitta, but too moist for kapha. Wheat's golden energy imbues cheerfulness and a positive outlook.

450 g (4 cups) wholemeal (whole-wheat) flour, plus extra for dusting

2 tablespoons sunflower oil

ghee, for brushing (see page 124)

Preparation time: 10 minutes
Cooking time: 25 minutes
Serves: 4

1 Mix the flour and oil together, and pour in enough hot water to make a soft, pliable dough. The more you knead it, the softer the bread will be.

2 Divide the dough into balls the size of a lime. Coat each one lightly with extra flour, and flatten out slightly.

3 Roll out on a floured surface into very flat discs about 10 cm (4 in) in diameter.

4 Heat a griddle or nonstick frying pan or skillet, and cook one flatbread until the surface appears bubbly. Turn over and cook the other side, pressing down lightly with a clean kitchen cloth to cook evenly. The bread is done when brown spots start to appear. Brush with ghee and keep warm.

5 Cook all the breads in a similar manner.

6 Serve hot.

ROTI

Potato-stuffed Bread

When eaten in moderation, carbohydrates such as wheat flour keep energy levels even and constant. A note about salt: ayurveda advises caution in the use of salt, as it causes weakness and lethargy, and can aggravate high blood pressure if eaten in large amounts. It does reduce vata, but too much can aggravate pitta and kapha.

450 g (4 cups) wholemeal (whole-wheat) flour

about 6 tablespoons sunflower oil

sea salt

POTATO FILLING

3 medium potatoes, about 300 g (10 oz)

1 tablespoon sunflower oil

½ teaspoon cumin seed

¼ teaspoon finely chopped fresh green chilli

½ teaspoon ground turmeric

sea salt

2 tablespoons finely chopped coriander (cilantro) leaves

Preparation time: 20 minutes
Cooking time: 45 minutes
Serves: 4

1 Boil the potatoes whole until cooked. Peel and mash.

2 Heat the oil in a heavy pan until almost smoking, and fry the cumin seed until dark. Add the chilli, turmeric and salt to taste.

3 Mix in the mashed potato and coriander. Set aside.

4 To make the dough, combine the flour, 2 tablespoons of the oil, a little salt and just enough water to combine. Knead until smooth and firm.

5 Divide the dough into 16 equal-sized balls. Roll each one out, dusting with a little flour if sticky, into a flat round about 8 cm (3 in) in diameter.

6 Smear a layer of the potato mixture over one disc, then place another rolled-out disc of dough over the top. Seal the edges to make a parcel, or paratha.

7 Heat a frying pan and dot with oil. Cook the parcels until tiny dark spots appear on the underside. Turn over and cook the other side.

8 Smear the entire bread with a little oil, and lift out onto a warmed platter. Keep warm while you cook the rest of the breads in a similar manner.

9 This bread is a meal in itself when eaten with natural (plain) yoghurt and hot mango pickle.

Semolina Pancakes

Semolina is cool in potency and sweet in 'rasa', or taste. In India it is often used as a restorative food, for everyone from children to the elderly. However, wheat sensitivity can be a problem, symptoms of this including headaches, lethargy and body aches. Food intolerances or allergies often arise because the body is not capable of handling the digestion of a particular food and produces antibodies instead. Many allergies can be overcome by simply avoiding particular foods in the long term.

150 g (1 cup) semolina

1 fresh green chilli, minced

handful of fresh coriander (cilantro) leaves, chopped

1 medium tomato, chopped

¼ teaspoon ground turmeric

1 tablespoon rice flour

a little sea salt

sunflower oil for shallow-frying

Preparation time: **10 minutes**
Cooking time: **30 minutes**
Serves: **4**

1 Combine all the ingredients except the oil in a mixing bowl. Pour in just enough cold water to make a thick batter and beat well.

2 Heat a heavy griddle and brush with oil. When the oil is nearly smoking, pour a large spoonful of batter in the centre of the griddle and quickly spread it into a thin disc using the back of the spoon or ladle. Allow to cook for a couple of minutes, then flip over to cook the other side. Dot the edges with a little more oil.

3 Continue in a similar manner until all the batter is used.

4 Serve the pancakes warm, with a vegetable curry such as Cauliflower with Coconut (see page 63).

RAVA DOSA

Millet Bread

This is a chunky, country-style bread that is especially recommended for people who are allergic to wheat. Millet is hot, light and dry, and therefore ideal for kapha. It also works on the body's insulin mechanism, helping kapha to digest starches better. Pitta is pacified by its inherent sweetness, while vata must combine it with a moist accompaniment to be able to tolerate it. The dryness of millet makes it more difficult to digest. For this reason, it needs to be eaten with something spicy and juicy.

225 g (2 cups) millet flour

butter or ghee (see page 124) for brushing

Preparation time: **10 minutes**
Cooking time: **25 minutes**
Serves: **4**

BAJRE

KI

BHAKRI

1 Put the flour into a large mixing bowl, make a well in the centre and pour in just enough water to make a soft, flaky dough.

2 Knead slightly, then divide the dough into 4 even-sized balls. Wet your palms and pat each down into a flat disc. You will need to keep wetting your palm so that the disc does not break into bits.

3 Heat a griddle until very hot, and brush with butter. Gently lift a disc of dough and place it on the griddle. Cook for 3-4 minutes, then carefully flip over to cook the other side. Next move the griddle off the heat and cook the disc directly over the flame or heat source for a few seconds each side, holding it with a pair of tongs - it should have firmed up by this time.

4 Brush with a little more butter and serve at once. This bread must be eaten very hot, as it becomes hard and slightly bitter on keeping.

Cornbread

This golden-coloured bread is eaten in Punjab as the first winter mists roll in with the promise of colder weather. Cornflour (cornstarch) and cornmeal are dry and warm, with sweet and astringent tastes, and they are beautifully balancing to kapha. Pitta and vata find them acceptable when they are moistened as in this recipe. Corn has been known to soothe an irritable bladder and is used to complement the treatment of kidney stones.

250 g (1½ cups) coarse cornmeal

pinch of sea salt

cornflour (cornstarch) for dusting

Preparation time: **10 minutes**
Cooking time: **30 minutes**
Serves: **4**

1 Make a stiff dough by adding enough water to the cornmeal and salt to combine. Knead until smooth, then form into 12 even-sized balls.

2 Place one on a floured surface, and pat with your palm to flatten it into a disc 10–12 cm (4–5 in) in diameter. Dust your palms with a little cornflour if necessary.

3 Heat a griddle until very hot, then gently lift the disc onto it. When the surface appears bubbly, turn over and cook on the other side. The bread is cooked when the surface is flecked with brown spots.

4 Serve hot, with a moist vegetable dish such as Spinach with Cottage Cheese (see page 64) or Okra in a Velvet Buttermilk Sauce (see page 69).

MAKAI

KI ROTI

Mung Bean Pancakes

The heat in green chillies depends on the amount of capsaicin present in the seeds, veins and skin. Chillies are indispensable in India; they actually help to cool the body during the scorching summers by dilating the blood vessels to increase circulation and promote perspiration. They also stimulate agni and are perfect for kapha and, in small doses, vata. They aggravate pitta too much and are best avoided if you are this constitutional type. The seeds are the hottest part, but removing them carefully will reduce the fieriness.

225 g (8 oz) dried mung beans, soaked overnight in cold water

1 fresh green chilli, minced

1 tablespoon freshly chopped coriander (cilantro) leaves

sea salt

ghee for brushing (see page 124)

Preparation time: 10 minutes plus overnight soaking
Cooking time: 20 minutes
Serves: 4

1 Drain the soaked mung beans and rinse well. Blend or process with a few teaspoonfuls of water.

2 Transfer to a deep mixing bowl and stir in enough water to make a thin, custard-like batter. Add the chilli, coriander and salt to taste.

3 Heat a griddle until very hot, and brush with ghee. Pour in a ladleful of batter and shape into a disc using the back of the ladle – you will need to do this quite quickly. When the surface bubbles, flip the pancake over and cook until golden. Continue cooking in a similar manner until all the batter has been used.

4 Serve the pancakes warm, with a chicken curry.

MUNG CHILLA

Salads & Raitas

Salads are fabulous for adding colour, texture and vitality to a meal, as long as they are not soaked in oil and fatty sauces. If you must use oil, choose olive oil, which is a monounsaturated fat beneficial in reducing cholesterol and keeping the heart healthy. It also contains natural antioxidants such as vitamin E, which is anti-ageing.

Raitas are cool and mild in taste and therefore bring balance to a meal, particularly if the dishes are highly spiced or fiery. They can include a combination of vegetables, fruit or flour dumplings and lightly spiced yoghurt, and they are often served chilled.

Cucumber & Dill Salad

Cucumbers are native to India and have been grown there for the past 3000 years. They have little nutritive value, but provide ample juice that is quenching in the parching heat. Cucumbers reduce pitta and vata, but increase kapha. Dill is not only a perfect complement to cucumber, but is also well known for its ability to prevent stomach disorders.

250 g (8 oz) cucumber, very finely chopped

½ teaspoon freshly chopped green chilli

2 tablespoons freshly chopped dill leaves

4 tablespoons desiccated (shredded) coconut

1 teaspoon sunflower oil

½ teaspoon black mustard seed

8 curry leaves

sea salt to taste

pinch of granulated sugar

Preparation time: 15 minutes
Cooking time: Nil
Serves: 4

1 Mix the cucumber, chilli, dill and coconut in a bowl.

2 Heat the oil until almost smoking in a small saucepan, and add the mustard seed.

3 When the seeds being to crackle, add the curry leaves and stir for a few seconds, then pour over the top of the cucumber mixture.

4 Add salt to taste and the sugar just before serving.

SUWACHI

KHAMANG KAKDI

White Radish in Yoghurt

The long, slim white radish known as mooli or daikon is pungent in taste and hot in potency. It is very stimulating to agni and therefore very good for kapha. Vata, too, benefits from its warmth, if it is eaten in small amounts. Pitta, however, finds this radish too sharp and does not tolerate it well. Pungent tastes, in moderation, make us feel passionate and motivated. Mooli, especially, is rich in potassium, which helps to maintain the heart and can quickly become depleted in the body if you are overstressed either emotionally or physically.

300 ml (1¼ cups) natural (plain) yoghurt

¼ teaspoon chilli powder

sea salt

1 medium mooli (white radish), about 150 g (5 oz), peeled and grated

MOOLI KA RAITA

Preparation time: **10 minutes**
Cooking time: **Nil**
Serves: **4**

1 Put the yoghurt, chilli powder and salt to taste in a large mixing bowl, and whisk together.

2 Drain the mooli of any juices, and fold into the yoghurt. Transfer to a serving bowl and chill slightly before serving.

Carrot & Raisin Salad

Although there are definite advantages to crunching through lots of raw foods such as carrot and cucumber, many of us overlook the benefits of lightly cooking these very same vegetables. Steaming or boiling carrots breaks down the strong plant cell walls and releases valuable carotenoids, which are essential for keeping the skin, eyes and tissues healthy. Raw carrots are excellent for vata and kapha, while pitta can handle them occasionally. They are cooling in the short term, but have a heating long-term effect, so they aggravate pitta over time if consumed in excess. Their orange energy is reminiscent of a beautiful sunrise and is a great antidepressant.

4 large carrots, about 300 g (10 oz), peeled and grated

2 tablespoons raisins, soaked

sea salt

pinch of granulated sugar

2 tablespoons freshly chopped coriander (cilantro) leaves

Preparation time: **10 minutes**
Cooking time: **5 minutes**
Serves: **4**

1 Put the carrot in a medium saucepan and pour in just enough boiling water to cover. Bring to a rapid boil, then remove from the heat and drain.

2 Combine the carrot, raisins, salt to taste, sugar and coriander in a large mixing or serving bowl. Toss together and serve.

GAJAR

KA SALAD

Potato & Yoghurt Salad

I love to serve this golden salad with a spicy meat curry, as its blend of textures and flavours – waxy, creamy, sour and sweet – truly complements the richness of the main course. This salad is seasoned with various spices. Black pepper kindles agni and reduces gas. It is also rich in chromium, which helps the metabolism of blood sugar and therefore plays a part in preventing diabetes. Pepper is also believed to be diuretic and is used in many aphrodisiac potions. Peppercorns have an indigo colour ray, which helps in bringing a balanced harmony between an overactive mind and an understimulated body.

4 medium potatoes, about 300 g (10 oz), boiled in their skins

sea salt

150 ml (²⁄₃ cup) natural (plain) yoghurt

1 tablespoon honey

½ teaspoon roasted ground cumin*

½ teaspoon chilli powder

¼ teaspoon freshly ground black pepper

1 tablespoon freshly chopped coriander (cilantro) leaves

Preparation time: 10 minutes
Cooking time: 20 minutes
Serves: 4

1 Peel the potatoes and cut them into cubes, then place them in a serving bowl. Dust with a little salt.

2 Combine the yoghurt, honey, cumin, chilli powder and pepper in a mixing bowl, and drizzle over the potatoes.

3 Scatter the coriander over the top and serve.

* If you cannot buy roasted ground cumin, simply dry-roast ordinary ground cumin for a few minutes over medium heat in a clean frying pan or skillet.

DAHI ALOO CHAAT

Green Raita

A stifling summer's day can be made instantly more bearable by a chilled bowl of this fresh raita. It is perfect served with a lightly spiced meat or vegetable kebab and Flatbread (see page 100). Mint is cooling and calming, and balances all the doshas. You can use any kind of mint, as all the edible varieties possess similar properties. Coriander (cilantro) adds pure green power, which is symbolic of natural balance and healing.

bunch of fresh mint (about a cupful of leaves)

bunch of coriander (cilantro) (about a cupful of leaves)

1 fresh green chilli

2 cloves garlic

½ teaspoon freshly grated ginger

sea salt

pinch of granulated sugar

250 ml (1 cup) natural (plain) yoghurt, beaten

fresh mint, to garnish (optional)

Preparation time: **15 minutes**
Cooking time: **Nil**
Serves: **4**

1 Blend or process the mint, coriander, chilli, garlic and ginger until smooth.

2 Stir in the salt to taste, sugar and yoghurt. Garnish with a sprig of mint if desired, and serve chilled.

HARA RAITA

Pomegranate Seeds Tossed in Spices

The small, juicy seeds are the edible part of a pomegranate. Although it can be slightly astringent, pomegranate has a sweet taste (see page 9) and is one the best foods for pitta. It calms a system that has been battered by too much salt or sugar, or by sour foods. Kapha also benefits from this fruit, while vata is only slightly aggravated. It is an invaluable remedy for an upset stomach and is even used for children. This ruby-red fruit contains potassium, one of the nutrients required to maintain blood pressure, and vitamin A, which strengthens the eyes.

1 large pomegranate

pinch of rock salt

1 tablespoon freshly squeezed lemon juice

freshly ground black pepper

Preparation time: **15 minutes**
Cooking time: **Nil**
Serves: **4**

1 Slice open the pomegranate and remove its seeds, discarding the skin and the membranes between the clusters of seeds.

2 Combine the pomegranate seeds, salt, lemon juice and a few grinds of pepper in a serving bowl. Toss through.

3 Chill slightly and serve.

ANAAR
KA
CHAAT

Sweet & Sour Banana Salad

Bananas are most nutritious when they are allowed to ripen on the stem. Modern-day picking and storage often does not allow the nutrients to develop to their full potential. Bananas are good for toning the stomach and digestion, but are poor for kapha types. Avoid eating bananas when you have a cold or sore throat, as their cool potency can be quite aggravating.

2 large bananas

rock salt

¼ teaspoon chilli powder

¼ teaspoon roasted ground cumin*

1 tablespoon freshly squeezed lemon juice

Preparation time: **10 minutes**
Cooking time: **Nil**
Serves: **4**

1 Slice the bananas into a serving bowl. Add the remaining ingredients and toss lightly.

2 Serve slightly chilled with Flatbread (see page 100) and a spicy curry.

* If you cannot buy roasted ground cumin, simply dry-roast ordinary ground cumin for a few minutes over medium heat in a clean frying pan or skillet.

KELE KA
CHAAT

Lettuce, Grape & Mango Salad

Cool and moist, lettuce is ideal for kapha and pitta, but vata needs to add oil or dressing to be able to tolerate it. Romaine (cos) lettuce is one of the most nutritious of lettuces, with its high stores of folic acid and vitamin A. Sweet purple grapes are tridoshic when eaten in moderation, and they are cooling in potency. They are rich in vitamins A and C, are considered diuretic and mildly laxative, and are useful in calming a rough or scratchy throat. The green, purple and orange energies of this salad bring happy and calming thoughts.

1 head of cos (romaine) lettuce

handful of sweet purple grapes

1 fresh ripe mango, peeled and cubed

DRESSING

1 tablespoon freshly squeezed lemon juice

salt and freshly ground black pepper

1 tablespoon honey

2 tablespoons olive oil

1 tablespoon chopped coriander (cilantro) leaves

Preparation time: **15 minutes**
Cooking time: **Nil**
Serves: **4**

1 Tear the lettuce into a serving bowl. Add the grapes and mango.

2 In a separate bowl, combine all the ingredients for the dressing, then drizzle over the salad.

3 Toss lightly and serve.

ANGOOR AUR AAM KA SALAD

Ginger Raita

Fresh ginger juice is wonderful for relieving coughs and colds. Ginger itself helps to dispel gas, improves digestion, boosts circulation and discourages inertia. In ayurveda it is referred to as 'maha aushadhi', or great medicine. A Sanskrit verse compares ginger to a lion and minor ailments to small animals who disappear when the lion arrives on the scene. Peel ginger only lightly; the essential oil to which it owes its efficacy lies just beneath the skin. Pitta should avoid ginger, while kapha does better with the dried version. Ginger's red energy is sure to put vitality into your day.

1 teaspoon sunflower oil

1 fresh green chilli

2 tablespoons grated fresh ginger

4 tablespoons shredded fresh coconut or desiccated (shredded) coconut

sea salt

150 ml (²⁄₃ cup) natural (plain) yoghurt, beaten

1 tablespoon raisins

Preparation time: **15 minutes**
Cooking time: **2 minutes**
Serves: **4**

1 Heat the oil until almost smoking in a heavy pan, and fry the chilli and ginger lightly. Blend or process with the coconut and salt to taste until smooth.

2 Beat the coconut mixture into the yoghurt and add the raisins.

3 Serve slightly chilled.

PACHADI

Tropical Pineapple & Coconut Salad

Sweet yellow pineapple is full of nutrients, most especially bromelain, which is excellent for the pancreas. Bromelain appears to be destroyed during cooking, however, so canned pineapple does not contain it. Pineapple is also rich in vitamin A, which helps the immune system. Pineapples have been used to calm gastritis and to tone the nervous system. Vata and pitta are happy with sweet, ripe pineapples, while kapha can manage only small amounts. Here it is combined with cooling coconut, which is soothing and a mild laxative.

150 g (about 3 cups) shredded coconut

2 tablespoons jaggery or soft brown sugar

2 dried red chillies, torn and soaked in water for 5 minutes

½ teaspoon mustard seed

sea salt

150 g (5 oz) ripe fresh pineapple, cubed

Preparation time: **20 minutes**
Cooking time: **Nil**
Serves: **4**

1 Blend or process the coconut, jaggery, chillies, mustard seed and a little salt to a coarse paste with a couple of teaspoonfuls of water.

2 Fold the pineapple pieces into the mixture.

3 Serve slightly chilled.

ANANAS

SASAM

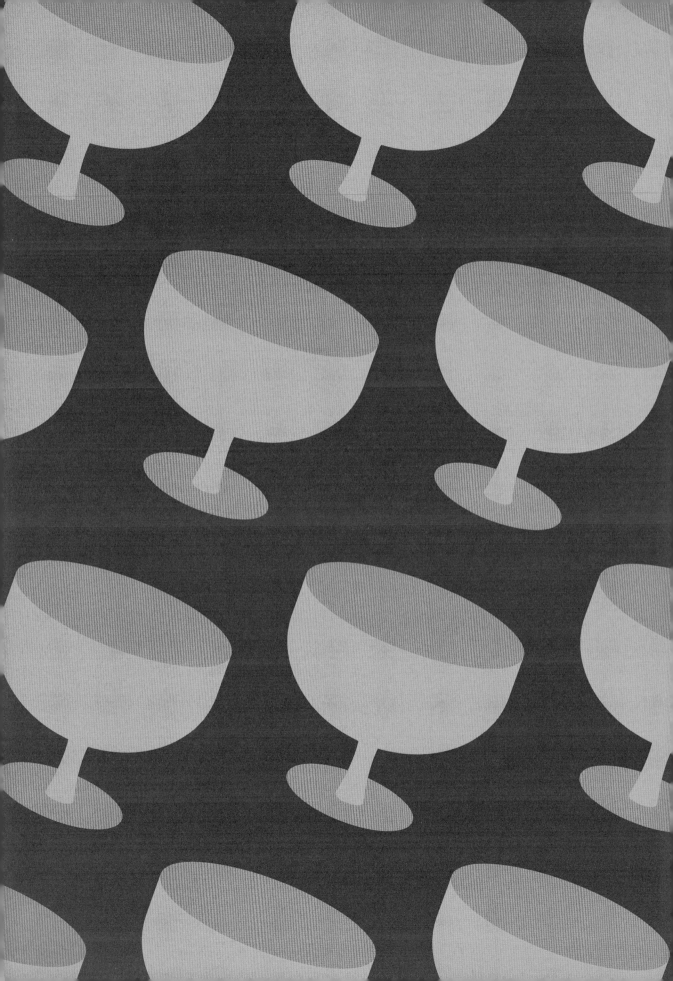

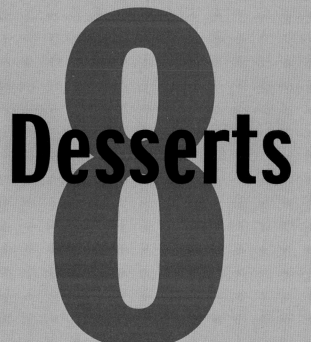

Desserts

India has a great tradition of puddings and desserts that are mainly used to celebrate an endless procession of festivals. Sweets are offered to the gods as holy foods and, as such, most are rich and heavy. Of course, a plethora of readily available fruit also means that light, natural sweets and desserts abound.

This is just as well, as ayurveda really does not recommend eating heavy desserts after a meal and cautions us against eating too many sweet things during the day as well. Common sense also tells us that this is inadvisable as rich sweets are difficult to digest, create toxins ('ama') and can add weight. If you do want to end your meal with dessert, it is best to finish off with something light, about half an hour after you have finished your main meal.

Stewed Prunes with Cream

Prunes are a wonderful source of iron and can boost a sluggish circulation. In ayurveda they are considered warm and laxative, so they are very good for expectant mothers as well. As prunes promote elimination, they are especially beneficial in the winter to kapha, as they help to relieve coughs and colds. Indigo foods such as prunes free the mind of fear and inhibition, and help to create confidence.

300 g (10 oz) pitted prunes

4 tablespoons sugar

4 tablespoons double (heavy) cream

2 tablespoons crushed almonds

2 sheets edible silver foil, to garnish (optional)

Preparation time: **10 minutes**
Cooking time: **15 minutes**
Serves: **4**

1 Put the prunes and 300 ml (1¼ cups) water in a saucepan, and stew over a low heat until soft and mushy. Add the sugar and stir.

2 Once the sugar has dissolved completely, spoon the mixture into serving bowls. Drizzle double cream over the fruit. Sprinkle the almonds over the top and decorate with a twist of silver foil, if using.

3 Serve slightly chilled.

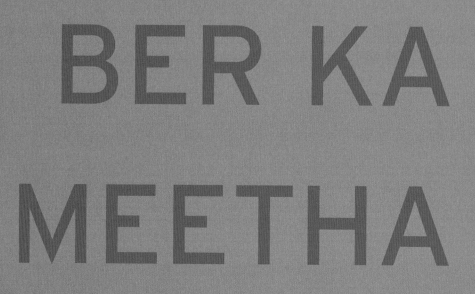

BER KA
MEETHA

Sesame Crackle

Sesame seed sweets are a winter delicacy in India because of their warm, lubricating properties. They are rather heavy to digest, so this dessert is best eaten in small amounts. Vata finds that sesame seeds provide the warmth to digest foods such as legumes better, whereas pitta and kapha are aggravated by this very quality. Sesame oil contains an antioxidant and therefore has anti-ageing properties. The golden energy of sesame brings cheerfulness to a cold, bleak day.

225 g (8 oz) white sesame seeds

225 g (1⅓ cups) crushed jaggery

pinch of ground cardamom

ghee for greasing (see page 124)

Preparation time: 10 minutes plus 1 hour
   for soaking
Cooking time: 35 minutes
Serves: 4

1 Wash the sesame seeds and soak in water for about an hour. Dry the seeds on a clean kitchen towel and lightly toast on a griddle or in a dry pan over a low heat. When they turn golden, remove to a dish to cool.

2 Put the jaggery and 300 ml (1¼ cups) water in a heavy saucepan, and bring to a boil. Reduce the heat and cook until it melts to a syrupy consistency, about 25 minutes. Remove from the heat.

3 Mix in the sesame seeds and cardamom, and stir through well.

4 Grease a large, flat plate with ghee and spread the sesame mixture thinly over it. Allow it to cool completely, then break it up or cut into diamonds. Leftover crackle can be stored in an airtight jar for up to 2 weeks.

TIL KI

CHIKKI

Rice & Nutmeg Pudding

In India this sweet is offered to the gods. The nutmeg that flavours it is widely used to cure poor digestion, as an aphrodisiac and as a remedy for insomnia. Nutmeg is well tolerated by vata, but pitta and kapha find it aggravating and should substitute an equal amount of cardamom in this recipe. The other flavouring, saffron, is also believed to be an aphrodisiac, and its mention can be found in ancient Indian romantic literature. It has been used to relieve melancholia, no doubt because of its vibrant orange energy. Saffron is cooling, toning and balancing to all the doshas.

150 g (1 cup) basmati rice, rinsed and drained

600 ml (2 ½ cups) milk

300 ml (1 ½ cups) evaporated milk

sugar or honey to taste

¼ teaspoon ground nutmeg

a few saffron threads

2 tablespoons sliced almonds

2 tablespoons raisins, soaked in water

Preparation time: 15 minutes
Cooking time: 1 hour 15 minutes
Serves: 4

1 Bring the rice and milk to a boil in a heavy saucepan, then simmer for about an hour over a very low heat until the rice is mushy. Mash it further with the back of a spoon.

2 Pour in the evaporated milk and sugar. Stir in the nutmeg and saffron, and cook for another 10 minutes.

3 Stir in the almonds and drained raisins.

4 Serve hot in winter or slightly chilled in summer.

PAL PAYASAM

Fresh Fruit Salad

Fruits are cleansing and rid the body of toxins. They are also amazingly easy to digest. For this they need to be eaten on their own or before a meal. Eaten after a heavy meal they sit on top of everything else in the stomach and are last in line to be digested. As they wait their turn, fermentation begins and gas is formed. If you eat them as a pudding, wait a while to give your digestion a chance to work on the main meal first. Also, fruits are healing only when they are naturally ripened and free of chemicals. Look for organically grown fruits or grow your own to make sure that you are not eating a load of chemicals as well. Add your favourite fruits here to make it special. Apples are cool and light, while pears, from the same family, are heavier and dry. Both, along with strawberries, apricots, peaches, cherries, plums and raspberries, are well suited to pitta and kapha. Vata thrives on fruits such as papaya, melons, bananas and citrus.

300 g (10 oz) fresh fruit (choose your favourite combination), peeled and cubed

honey to taste

1 tablespoon freshly squeezed lemon juice

2 tablespoons freshly chopped mint leaves

Preparation time: **15 minutes**
Cooking time: **Nil**
Serves: **4**

1 Combine the fruit in a mixing bowl.

2 Make a dressing with the honey, lemon juice and mint, and drizzle over the fruit. Toss lightly.

3 Transfer the salad to a serving bowl, and serve slightly chilled.

PHALON KA

SANGAM

Sweet Flour Balls

These sweets, flavoured with cardamom, deliver the benefits of ghee (clarified butter). One of ayurveda's elixirs, ghee is the pure form of butter fat. It is often used as a base for herbal medicines, as it aids the absorption of the nutrients with which it is mixed. Every Indian home has a store of ghee - it is sweet, cool and light. Also, in reasonable amounts, it is rejuvenating and a tonic. Ghee is eaten in winter to lubricate dry, flaky skin. It is available commercially, but is really very easy to make yourself if you have the time (see below).

50 g (2 oz) ghee*

225 g (2 cups) besan (chickpea flour)

1 tablespoon milk

¼ teaspoon ground cardamom

1 tablespoon raisins

Preparation time: **10 minutes**
Cooking time: **30 minutes**
Serves: **4**

1 Heat the ghee in a heavy saucepan and add the flour. Cook, stirring continuously, until the flour mixture turns coppery in colour and is aromatic.

2 Remove from the heat and sprinkle the milk over the top. Leave uncovered to cool. When almost cool, add the cardamom and raisins.

3 Scoop small handfuls of the mixture in your palm and press into balls the size of a small lime.

4 Serve cold. Any remaining balls can be stored in an airtight container for several days.

* To make your own ghee, melt unsalted butter over a gentle heat, skimming off and discarding the foam that forms on top and cooking the butter until it turns golden. Insufficient cooking will lead to mould forming during storing. Use immediately or wrap well and refrigerate for up to six months.

BESAN
KE
LADDOO

Oranges in Clotted Milk

Ayurveda has always recognized the light, cooling and nourishing properties of cow's milk. However, it also recommends that it be served hot and warmed with spices such as cardamom or cinnamon to make it balancing, rather than aggravating. Oranges are best for vata and are known to purify the blood, stimulate agni and tone the liver. They are beneficial in their postdigestive effect (see page 9), and sweet and cooling, so they make a delicious summer dessert. The orange energy of the fruit adds to the optimism of the season.

600 ml (2 ½ cups) milk

raw cane sugar to taste

¼ teaspoon ground cardamom

½ teaspoon saffron threads

150 g (5 oz) orange segments, skinned and seeded

sliced almonds, to garnish (optional)

Preparation time: 10 minutes
Cooking time: 1 hour
Serves: 4

1 Pour the milk into a heavy-bottomed saucepan and bring to a boil. Reduce the heat and simmer until the volume has reduced by half, about 30 minutes.

2 Add the sugar and continue cooking for another 15 minutes or until the mixture is thick and creamy.

3 Remove from the heat and cool completely. Sprinkle in the cardamom and saffron, and add the orange segments. Chill slightly.

4 Spoon into individual serving glasses and serve topped with a few sliced almonds, if using.

NARANGI RABDI

Pistachio Cream

This rather rich dessert is smooth and creamy, and beautifully flavoured with pistachios, which are known to provide energy when your resources are low. They are best for vata, as kapha and pitta may find them too heavy and oily. However, ayurveda considers pistachios to be restorative and warm, and suggests eating them to tonify the system. The honey in this dessert is extremely healing, but is quite volatile and breaks down in the presence of heat. It is best to use it cool or at the very last moment. Young, fresh honey is most healing, especially for pitta.

1.2 litres (5 cups) thick, Greek-style yoghurt

1 teaspoon saffron threads, soaked in 1 teaspoon milk

honey to taste

½ teaspoon ground cardamom

3 tablespoons crushed pistachio nuts

Preparation time: 20 minutes plus overnight draining
Cooking time: Nil
Serves: 4

1 Tie the yoghurt in a clean kitchen cloth or cheesecloth, and hang up overnight to drain away the whey.

2 The following day, put the drained yoghurt in a large mixing bowl. Stir in the saffron with the milk, honey and cardamom. Whisk together until fluffy, about 5 minutes.

3 Mix in half the pistachios and spoon into individual serving bowls.

4 Serve slightly chilled, sprinkled with the remaining pistachios.

PISTA KA
SHRIKHAND

Date & Carrot Halwa

Ayurvedic texts speak very highly of dates. They are calming for vata and pitta, but aggravate kapha. Fresh dates are heating, whereas the dried ones lose this quality and become quite mild. Dates fortify the liver so are a good antidote for lovers of alcohol. They also help to neutralize bladder inflammations and fevers brought on by cold weather. Here they are combined with blood-purifying carrots. The orange energy of this dessert will boost the sex drive as well as encourage enthusiasm and optimism.

2 tablespoons ghee (see page 124)

150 g (5 oz) carrots, grated

150 g (5 oz) dried dates, pitted and chopped

granulated sugar to taste

300 ml (1¼ cups) milk

½ teaspoon ground cardamom

edible silver foil, to decorate (optional)

Preparation time: **15 minutes**
Cooking time: **20 minutes**
Serves: **4**

1 Heat the ghee until almost smoking in a heavy-bottomed pan, and fry the carrot, stirring occasionally to prevent sticking.

2 When the carrot is translucent, add the dates and sugar, and stir until blended.

3 Pour in the milk, reduce the heat and cook until the carrot and dates are mushy and the milk has been absorbed.

4 Remove from the heat and mix in the cardamom.

5 Serve warm, decorated with silver foil, if using.

KHAJOOR

GAJAR KA HALWA

Spiced Semolina & Nut Halwa

This is a special sweet, given to people who need great reserves of energy such as athletes or new mothers. Its golden-yellow energy ray acts like a tonic, fortifying and balancing the system. Whole wheats, and therefore semolina, are considered cooling, and this makes a wonderful summer dessert to counteract enervating heat. When served warm and spiced as in this recipe, semolina becomes appropriate for all seasons, most especially for vata and pitta. Kapha is aggravated by wheat, so this can only be an occasional treat.

3 teaspoons ghee (see page 124)

150 g (1 cup) semolina

granulated sugar to taste

300 ml (1¼ cups) warm water or milk

½ teaspoon ground cardamom

1 teaspoon rosewater

Preparation time: **5 minutes**
Cooking time: **15 minutes**
Serves: **4**

1 Put the ghee and semolina in a heavy-bottomed saucepan and cook until the mixture becomes golden and aromatic.

2 Add the sugar and stir for a minute. Reduce the heat and pour in the water or milk. Stir rapidly to prevent lumps forming as it thickens. Continue stirring until the sugar has dissolved and the semolina is soft and fluffy. Remove from the heat.

3 Stir in the cardamom and rosewater, and serve warm. You can press or cut the halwa into shapes if desired.

SOOJI KA HALWA

Sweet Rice

The repertoire of ayurvedic nutrition contains an endless variety of nourishing stews made with grains. Modern research has also found that eating a good daily portion of grains raises the level of the amino acid tryptophan in the brain a couple of hours after ingestion. With the help of tryptophan the brain makes, among other substances, a compound called serotonin, which makes us feel calm and satisfied. This recipe works well for all the doshas. In South India it is made as a traditional offering to the sun during the annual harvest festival.

150 g (1 cup) basmati rice, rinsed and drained

3 tablespoons mung dal (split mung beans), rinsed and drained

pinch of salt

425 ml (1¾ cups) hot water, plus extra 150 ml (⅔ cup)

150 g (1 cup) soft brown sugar or jaggery

4 tablespoons ghee (see page 124)

2 tablespoons raw cashew nuts

2 tablespoons raisins

½ teaspoon ground cardamom

Preparation time: **10 minutes**
Cooking time: **40 minutes**
Serves: **4**

1 Put the rice, dal and salt in a heavy-bottomed saucepan along with 425 ml (1¾ cups) hot water. Bring to a boil, reduce the heat and simmer for about 20 minutes until soft and mushy. Remove from the heat and set aside.

2 In the meantime, mix the sugar with remaining 150 ml (⅔ cup) hot water and cook over a low heat until well dissolved.

3 Add this syrup to the cooked rice, and cook further until the liquid has been absorbed. Remove from the heat.

4 Heat the ghee until almost smoking in a small saucepan, and add the cashew nuts and raisins. Stir for a few seconds, then pour the entire mixture into the rice.

5 Stir in the cardamom and serve warm.

PONGAL

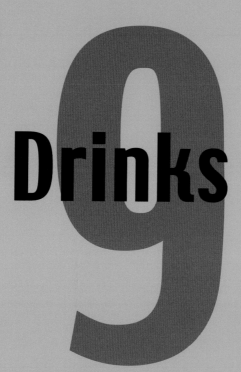

Drinks

9

Ayurveda suggests sipping a drink in moderation during a meal. Water at room temperature is best, as iced drinks only douse agni and inhibit digestion. Teas, juices and dairy-based drinks have all traditionally been used to stimulate or heal, depending on the circumstances. You can choose what suits you best as an accompaniment to a meal or as a drink before or after dinner.

Herbal drinks are simple to make and work effectively to keep the organs toned and working efficiently. Ayurveda does not consider alcohol to be unhealthy. In fact, many recipes for herbal wines exist in classic ayurvedic texts. As with all things, however, anything in excess is harmful, and pitta, especially, should be wary of drinking too much alcohol.

Hot Ginger Milk

This is one of the best drinks for vata, and kapha benefits, too, if cow's milk is replaced with goat's milk. Goat's milk produces less mucus than cow's milk and is helpful in conditions such as dysentery and diarrhoea. I would serve it to pitta people with a pinch of dry ginger instead of the fresh variety. Powdered, or ground, ginger is effective in dispelling gas.

600 ml (2 ½ cups) cow's milk or goat's milk

½ teaspoon grated fresh ginger or ¼ teaspoon ground ginger

sugar to taste

Preparation time: **5 minutes**
Cooking time: **20 minutes**
Serves: **4**

1 Boil the milk with the ginger in a heavy-bottomed saucepan. Reduce the heat, add sugar and simmer for 5 minutes.

2 Pour into individual cups and serve hot.

ADRAK
DOODH

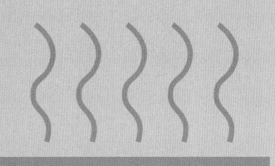

Spiced Digestive Tea

This is superb as an after-dinner digestive and helps to wash down the grease and spice of a meal. Fennel and cumin are known to promote good digestion. In India both are often boiled in water, strained out and the liquid given to even very tiny babies. Cardamom helps to lighten the effects of a heavy meal and settles the stomach. Coriander seeds have a slight peppery aroma and are pungent, yet they are cooling and tone the digestive system.

1 teaspoon fennel seed

1 teaspoon cumin seed

3 green cardamom pods, bruised

1 teaspoon coriander seed

600 ml (2 ½ cups) water

honey to taste

dash of milk (optional)

Preparation time: **5 minutes**
Cooking time: **15 minutes**
Serves: **4**

1 Put the spices in a heavy-bottomed saucepan and stir over a high heat for a couple of minutes until they begin to sizzle and change colour.

2 Pour the water in and bring to a boil. Reduce the heat and simmer for 10 minutes. The water will have turned golden.

3 Remove from the heat, strain and discard the spices.

4 Sweeten to taste with honey and serve hot. Vatas and pittas can add a dash of milk, if liked.

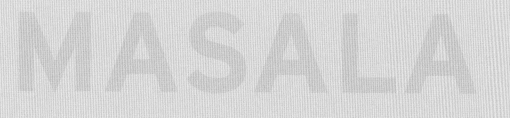

MASALA CHAI

Lemon Grass & Mint Tea

In India an assortment of herbs and spices are boiled in milk or water to make a wide variety of teas that are considered healthy and detoxifying. In this summer recipe lemon grass adds a sweet, lemony fragrance and helps to tone the kidneys and all the membranes of the body. The mint stimulates digestion and banishes gas. It is also used as a diuretic. This tea is calming to pitta and kapha, and neutralizes vata. The green energy of this fresh drink will also help to calm the body and mind.

600 ml (2 ½ cups) water

few sprigs of lemon grass

small handful of fresh mint leaves

honey to taste

Preparation time: **5 minutes**
Cooking time: **20 minutes**
Serves: **4**

1 Bring the water to a boil in a large saucepan. Add the lemon grass, reduce the heat and simmer for 5 minutes. Remove from the heat.

2 Add the mint leaves and steep for 10 minutes. Strain, discard the herbs, and add honey to taste.

3 Serve hot or cold.

PATTI KI CHAI

Fig & Turmeric Milk

This golden bedtime drink with a surprise at the bottom of the cup was a childhood favourite of mine. It was conjured up by my grandmother to relieve the often combined ills of a sore throat and constipation. Turmeric is highly respected for its antiseptic and anti-inflammatory action. It also strengthens the liver and is a wonderful blood purifier. Dried figs are nature's best laxative, yet most children will not need much persuasion to eat them. In this recipe they absorb the sweet honeyed milk and become fat and chewy. This drink is especially good for vata and pitta.

600 ml (2 ½ cups) cow's milk*

¼ teaspoon ground turmeric

8 dried figs

honey to taste

Preparation time: Nil
Cooking time: **10 minutes**
Serves: **4**

1 Pour the milk into a heavy-bottomed saucepan and add the turmeric and figs. Bring to a boil.

2 Remove from the heat. Take four cups or mugs, and put two figs at the bottom of each one. Pour the milk over the top and sweeten with honey.

3 Serve at once.

* Kapha types should substitute soya milk for the cow's milk.

ANJEER
DOODH

Tamarind Cooler

The people of Rajasthan have drunk this sweet and sour cooler to counteract the fierce desert heat for many years. This delicious recipe has now travelled all over the country and is widely served during the summer months. Tamarind is cooling and a superb aid to digestion. However, it is tolerated only by vata, as pitta types find it too fiery for their systems, while kapha people are aggravated by its tang.

2 tablespoons tamarind pulp

600 ml (2½ cups) water

½ teaspoon ground black pepper

½ teaspoon ground cardamom

rock salt to taste

raw cane sugar to taste

few sprigs of fresh mint leaves

Preparation time: 10 minutes
Cooking time: **Nil**
Serves: 4

1 Whisk together the tamarind pulp and a little of the water in a small bowl into a smooth paste. Stir into the remaining water.

2 Add the pepper, cardamom, salt and sugar. Mix well.

3 Serve slightly chilled, topped with mint.

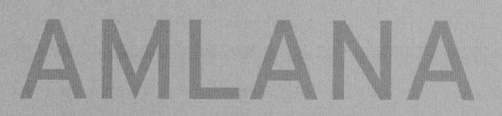

AMLANA

Minty Yoghurt Cooler

This refreshing green drink is a real thirst quencher and lifts the spirits. It goes well with a spicy main course, as it helps to neutralize the fiery effect of chillies and hot spices. It is good for vata, but pitta and kapha should avoid this drink or use soya yoghurt.

1 teaspoon cumin seed

handful of fresh mint leaves

handful of fresh coriander (cilantro) leaves

300 ml (1¼ cups) natural (plain) yoghurt

300 ml (1¼ cups) water

rock salt to taste

Preparation time: **15 minutes**
Cooking time: **Nil**
Serves: **4**

1 Dry-roast the cumin seed on a small griddle or skillet, then blend to a fine powder. Set aside.

2 Blend or process the mint and coriander to a fine paste.

3 Mix together the mint paste, yoghurt, water, salt and cumin powder in a large mixing bowl, and pour into individual serving glasses.

BOORANI

Carrot & Beetroot Juice

Vegetable juices have long been used in ayurvedic healing for specific ailments. They work best when drunk on an empty stomach. Carrot juice, which is rich in biotin as well as other nutrients, is here combined with beet juice, which contains folic acid and manganese. Biotin helps to maintain the skin, hair and nerves. Folic acid is known to affect mood, and manganese is associated with metabolism of fatty acids. This orange-red juice calms kapha and vata, but aggravates pitta. Thanks to its biotin content it is especially healing if you have a candida infection.

8 large juicy carrots, rinsed

3 large beetroot (red beets), peeled

Preparation time: **10 minutes**
Cooking time: **Nil**
Serves: **4**

1 Put the vegetables through a juicer, then strain.

2 Serve the juice at once.

GAJAR BEET KA RUS

Fresh Grape Juice

This light juice is suitable for all doshas, but only when you use grapes that are wholly sweet with no hint of astringency. Kapha types should drink it only in small quantities and well diluted. Purple grapes produce a healthier, more healing juice. I suggest you use organic grapes for this recipe, as this fruit especially is known to be liberally sprayed with chemicals in commercial vineyards. Grapes contain a high proportion of natural sugars, so diabetics should consult their doctor about eating them.

1 kg (2 lb) fresh, sweet, seedless purple grapes

Preparation time: 15 minutes
Cooking time: Nil
Serves: 4

1 Rinse the grapes well, then put them through a juicer.

2 Strain the liquid and serve at once.

ANGOOR
KA RUS

Soothing Herbal Tea

South Indians serve this healing tea throughout the day. The spices work to soothe and tone various organs and tissues, and the warmth of the drink calms the nerves and restores equilibrium. It is especially comforting if you have a cough, cold or the flu, but it also makes an exceptional everyday drink to keep the throat in good condition. Barley is diuretic and helps to calm an inflamed bladder. I always use organic barley to avoid consuming a load of toxins.

3 tablespoons organic barley

½ teaspoon cracked black peppercorns

½ teaspoon ground cardamom

3 cloves, bruised

½ teaspoon ground ginger

500 ml (2 cups) water

2 tablespoons milk (or soya milk for kapha)

jaggery or raw cane sugar to taste

Preparation time: **5 minutes**
Cooking time: **15 minutes**
Serves: **4**

1 Put the barley, peppercorns, cardamom, cloves, ginger and water in a large saucepan, and bring to a boil.

2 Reduce the heat and simmer for 10 minutes. Strain, then add the milk and jaggery.

3 Serve hot.

KASHAYA

Nutty Milk

Indian weddings are replete with ribaldry and innuendo, and the nuptial chamber is decorated with flowers and perfumed sheets. A glass of this nutty milk is strategically placed beside the bed, as it is believed to provide the new husband with vigour, energy and staying power. For these very reasons it is also favoured by athletes, dancers or those in physically demanding occupations. Walnuts are considered aphrodisiac in effect, pistachios provide energy and almonds, which are the most beneficial of all the nuts, nourish the entire system.

2 tablespoons whole blanched almonds

2 tablespoons whole blanched pistachio nuts

1 tablespoon whole walnuts

600 ml (2½ cups) milk*

honey to taste

Preparation time: 15 minutes
Cooking time: Nil
Serves: 4

1 Blend or process the almonds, pistachios and walnuts to a fine paste with a little of the milk.

2 Stir the paste into the remaining milk and sweeten to taste.

3 Serve at room temperature.

* This recipe is best for vata. Kapha and pitta will benefit by using soya milk instead of cow's milk.

SUHANA

DOODH

Index

Acknowledgements

This book would not have been possible without the help of many people over many years. First, a big thank you to my grandmother who brought me up with an innate sense of what is healthy eating, based on centuries of ayurvedic wisdom. Also, a *namaste* to the many teachers who guided me on how holistic nutrition can be applied to a changing way of life. Also hearty thanks to my agent Teresa Chris for her support, to Judith More and to Lisa Dyer at Carlton for their enthusiasm, and to Siobhan O'Connor for her wonderful editing.